Introduction

Hello, my name is Norrms and I live in a beautiful part of the UK called in Torquay in Devon with my long suffering wife and "Angel" Elaine. Most of our grandchildren also live around here which is great. Four years ago I was diagnosed with Alzheimer's and from then on I have dedicated my life to raising awareness about this awful disease.

I have decided to call this book SILENT VOICES (my battle with Alzheimer's continues) because I wrote a poem called Silent Voices for World Alzheimer's Day last year and I was lucky enough to have it read out at Gloucestershire Cathedral on the Night of W.A Day.

This book has no frilly bits, no nice pictures ECT but was it does have is Truth, Honesty and a passion for not only beating this awful disease but reducing the Stigma that always accompanies it. Please enjoy and God Bless each and every one of you

Norrms

1

Dedications

I would like to dedicate this book as always to my wonderful family and also my fantastic friends around the world who have not only supported me through thick and thin but have always been there for me at my very worst times.

I would also like to give a great mention to my friend "Across the Pond" in the states Stan Goldberg, who is not only an International award winning Author himself, but a wonderful Editor himself. Thank you Stan.

I also couldn't forget my wonderful friend Lori le Bay for the "Alzheimer's Speaks" website who has helped me enormously spreading awareness not only through her Site but also on American Radio.

SILENT VOICES

Silent voices shouting everywhere

Silent, yet still rising through the air,

Eyes that look but do not see,

Beating heart inside of me,

Forever wanting their life back,

No more wandering this lonely track,

To talk, to laugh, be understood,

To live their lives as they should,

One year there, next year gone,

Like the setting of the sun,

The Dementia Demon comes along,

Takes away your favourite song,

I have all this yet to come,

Vacant stare, body numb,

But to the end and from the start,

Place your hand around my heart,

Feel it beat inside of me,

Look in my eyes and you will see,

Happy scenes without a tear,

And my silent voice you will hear

INDEX

A Christmas Wish

Well, it's that time of year again and I have just been looking back on my computer and in my documents to see what I have been up to!!
PHEW!! It's been quite a year by all accounts!! Something`s I still remember, like the victory we had with BUPA and changing their wording on their documents. Also seeing our very own Memory cafe on the BBC news and talked about on Radio Devon. Highlights of the year has to be going to the Dementia Uk conference in Bournemouth and going home to my home town of Bolton to speak at the carer`s conference, I was so proud to be asked !! There are so many other things I have just seen so there are far too many to mention, I would be here all day!!LOL

The very low point of this year was the untimely death of my wonderful mother in June. I still hear her sometimes calling my name, is that the Alzheimer's or just wishful thinking? I don't really care what it is; it's so nice to hear her sometimes. I still miss her so much and if ever a hero walked this earth it was she. The one thing that does stand out more than anything else is the amount of dear, honest and supportive friends I have made over the last twelve months. It is well documented with me that when I was first diagnosed with Alzheimer's three years ago I lost 70% of my "so called friends" I can honestly say I have more than doubled than now in honest genuine friends, who accept me for who I am and only see me and not the illness. This is the most precious gift I have ever had (Apart from my "Angel wife Elaine and children) and for that I will forever thankful to you all. Sometimes I try not to look too far into the future for reasons I am sure you will understand but what I do look forward to is continuing these friendships I have made for a very long time to come. Each and every one of you holds a place in my heart which will never be diminished. As for my wish for next year? Well, a cure would be nice!! But failing that I just hope that each and every one of us touched by this awful illness will be able to understand it a little better and deal with it as it happens. I hope that the Stigma of this disease will be reduced so much it will disappear and Dementia will be talked about openly and honestly so all will understand how important this is to so many people. I hope that there will be a way to diagnose this illness as early as possible so to give people the chance to do what they always wanted to do and spend that precious time with their loved ones and friends enjoying every moment of it. I hope that all my friends and their friends find the strength and courage to fight this disease with everything they have.
Most of all I hope to be a part of all the above hopes by raising my voice about it at every opportunity, raising awareness as much as I can and hopefully being there on the day someone announcer's a cure!!

Alzheimer`s On Christmas Day

I have nine grandchildren, two of which live in Australia, one who still lives in the north of England, and six who were in the same front room as me on Christmas day. Can you imagine how hard it is sitting there watching your grandchildren, both young and old run riot, when you know that there is such a good chance you are going to forget all of these happy faces ? I have absolutely no memory of last Christmas so being sat there wondering how long it would be before I forget this one was one of the most emotional times I have ever sat through. The sheer enormity of the situation runs through your bones like shockwaves!! I sat there, trying to smile through complete anguish whilst trying to answer a million questions at once from my darling little ones. It was grandad this? Grandad that? And I have trouble keeping up at the best of times!!LOLL but through all this, all I saw was their smiles and their hopes in their eyes, I could almost feel their future mapping out in front of them, so much to look forward too, so much to do and so much to SAY!!! LOLL Just then, a hand slipped into mine and when I turned it was my "Angel" Elaine who always seemed to know when I was struggling a little bit. She gently squeezed my hand and smiled at me just at the point where I thought I was going to collapse into a heap, sobbing and upset. I smiled back and nodded at her, saying in my small way I had just caught up with myself and was ok for the time being. Elaine is my tower of strength and without her and my family I wouldn't have the courage to do what I do now. When you have been diagnosed with Dementia/Alzheimer's you don't think about Christmases, weddings, births ECT, in fact you don't think about much at first because your mind is in such turmoil. Being diagnosed with early onset and knowing you have it can be a curse as well as a blessing. The blessing is that you can spend precious time with your loved ones and your friends, you can cherish every moment of the day, and in my case I can continue to raise awareness to this awful disease and hopefully be around when the stigma that goes with it is totally eradicated and a cure found.

The curse is knowing you have it, which is sometime's just as bad as having Alzheimer's. Along my travels in life I have met someone who had a brain tumour and survived. I have met a few who have been diagnosed with Cancer and now look the picture of health. I myself 16 months ago had to have an operation for a serious Hernia which had its complications. The surgeon told my wife Elaine and me just before I went to the operating table that I had less than a 10% chance of survival because of my heart problems so if we needed to say anything now would be a good time, I survived!! But!! I have never met ANYBODY YET who has survived Alzheimer`s!!! NOT ONE SINGLE SOUL!!! Can you imagine the frustration that runs through me when you hear of certain medical bodies who will not put patient before cost??? Can you imagine the frustration at knowing that millions still think its and elderly disease and not a disease of the brain? All these things and more just give me the drive and determination to change things. But most of all, the thing that drives me forward more than anything is the look of hope and expectation in my grandchildren's eyes!! The sheer innocence of what is yet to come and the longer we can keep that innocence in their eyes the better!! This is why a cure must be found and found soon. I don't want my grandchildren or anybody else's grandchildren going through the horrors of seeing their grandmothers of grandfathers succumbing to this horrendous disease. I mentioned earlier about never having met anybody who has survived this disease, and unfortunately that statement is 100%true, but I would like to introduce the first person who WILL Survive it, and that person will hopefully be yours truly, myself, and thousands of others who come after me.

The time has come now to raise our voices and make 2011 the year we all survive. Let's hope and pray this is the year that everybody who is connected in some way with this disease see`s an end to the turmoil and destruction this illness brings. We Must Live In Hope ,Where There Is Hope, There Is Life

It`s Christmas Time

Its Christmas time again, God bless you one and all,

We got through this year, together we stood tall,

We faced all our troubles, and we faced our fears,

Getting through the bad times, drying all the tears,

Laughing through the good times, helping here and there,

Showing all our courage, showing that we care,

So what of the future? What will next year bring?

What tune will we be whistling? So together we can sing,

About our hopes and dreams, and how we will succeed,

In beating the dementia demon, we will sow the seed,

For others that will follow, so no more sickness reigns,

And dementia`s demons, never call again.

Have a very merry Christmas and a happy new year,

SEASONS GREETINGS

A Merry Christmas to one and all,

From Elaine, the kids and me,

And a very happy new year,

From all here in Torquay,

The tree is up, the presents wrapped,

And there`s happiness all around,

When we go to bed on Christmas Eve,

We are waiting for that sound,

The sound of bells and reindeer hoofs,

As he quickly passes by,

And, then as if by magic,

There the presents lie,

Thank you Father Christmas,

Thanks for all you do,

And a very merry Christmas

To everyone of you

MERRY CHRISTMAS AND A HAPPY NEW YEAR

The Loneliest Time of the Year

Yesterday we has our last meeting of the Torbay Dementia leadership group before the Christmas break and it was such a good meeting with lots of things achieved and discussed. The main topic was how to identify and help people with Dementia who don't have a carer or loved one coming round to help, and as you probably know by now, this got me thinking. Christmas time can certainly be the loneliest time of the year for some people but for people with Dementia and their carer's, more so. Not only would I ask all who reads this to keep an eye out and your ears open for people who might just be struggling a little more at this time of year but also think about the effect that Dementia has on not only the people who have it but also their wonderful carer's and loved ones. On a personal basis as I have already written, it's hard to try and remember what has happened in the last year but even harder to think about what MIGHT happen in the next year!! This is the curse of my Alzheimer's!! I want to try and remember the past and cant!! And I really don't want to think about the future sometimes but some days it's all I worry about!! This must in my mind also affect many others who suffer from this terrible disease. I know ask myself "Will I still remember this Christmas? NO I can't remember last Christmas!!" "What will happen to me in the next 12 months? Only the big Fella knows that".

"Will this be the year I take a downturn because of my illness and the Alzheimer's starts to win this battle?" "No one knows " All these things and MORE go through my mind at this time of year, but I think it's so IMPORTANT to remember that Loved One`s and carer`s must be asking themselves the same thing??

"What will this year bring for my loved one?" "How quickly will he or she deteriorate?" How much more of my husband or wife or relation will I lose this year?? So this is the time I believe for us all to come together and promise each other next year will be better. This is the time to stand shoulder to shoulder and say

"Next Year Things Will be different!!"

"Next year people will listen to our voices and we will be heard"

And next year we will make the changes we want so we can see a huge improvement in the way Dementia is observed and dealt with. And I promise you all as I always do that I will try my best to be as instrumental as is humanly possible to be a part of this change. God Bless each and every one of you and a special thanks to all the carers and professionals who help in this fight for change.

Time Of Year

Hiya, well, it's that time of year again when we try to think about the year just gone and our hopes for the future. Now, the thing is, the future I can dream and hope for, but the Past!! That's a different kettle of fish altogether!! At this time of year most people are looking back at times gone past in the last year, their achievements, their happy times and sometimes unfortunately the sad times. Unfortunately because of the nature of the illness a person with Dementia can't do this, (As much as they want to) This is only what I can describe as one of the most frustrating things connected with this awful illness and no matter how hard I try, sometimes nothing comes. I sometimes think about my wonderful mum dying such a long time ago only to be reminded that it was only in June this year!! It hurts so much even now to be told that!! Something's I can remember things but it's all what I call very distorted and mixed up and my memories of places and happenings don't come easily. If anybody asks me what I would like for Christmas, my answer is always the same, I would like my memory back please!! But as I know, until a cure is found this isn't possible, so what can we all do to help?

In my humble opinion I would like to see people with dementia getting Photographs of the past years events, i.e., marriages, christenings, births and birthday parties ECT. Maybe put on some sort of Collage all wrapped up as a big present!! Also (In my case) popular music from the past year, recorded on a CD, or even better, in some cases, a recording of our children's/Grandchildren's voices to be played and hopefully remembered. All these things could jog the memory and bring back some wonderful memories for some of us, who knows?? It's just an idea of what I would like to get, it may work it may not but worth a try I think? It's because of all the hard work and dedication from all you carer's / loved one's and professionals out there that we are here today to celebrate and look forward to a happy Christmas and a good New Year. Without your love and commitment we wouldn't be here now!! That's the long and short of it!!

So on behalf of myself and every other person with Dementia I would just like to say, from the bottom of my heart, such a big THANK YOU!! For all you do and have done in the past year, and also the support you have given my family and myself over the past year had been overwhelming.

My Christmas wish?? That a cure will be found soon, or if not, I am hopefully granted more time on this earth to make changes for the betterment of others and continue my work to help people understand that we, as people with Dementia are still the same person inside and together, with your help, we can beat this thing!!!

My Battle With Alzheimer`s

As my battle with Alzheimer`s rages on, the conversation with (My Angel) Elaine in the car turns to how things have been lately and how well the medication has been working as I have now been taking Ebixa for fourteen months now. I sit in STUNNED silence as she explains that she has seen a small downturn in my well being, so the car is pulled over to a local beauty spot as I listen intensely. Elaine says that the last few weeks I have become very irritable and my favourite saying is "Why am I always wrong!!!?? Or "You didn't tell me that you must have imagined it!!" As I listen, small instances come flooding back as I can hear myself saying these things. I listen in absolute horror at some of the things I have said to my darling wife, the one who has backed me all the way through life and now has the task of looking after me full time whilst having the added worry of seeing me disappear right in front of her eyes, slowly but surely disappearing in body and mind. A lot of what I am being told I have no memory of and it's like Elaine is telling me a story about somebody else she has been told about. I shake my head in utter disbelief that I have behaved this way as anybody who knows me knows I am so laid back I am practically horizontal!!LOL

Then the thought hit me like a shot! Is this how denial of the illness starts? Do I start to argue with the only person I have ever loved about the daftest things but yet causing so much heartache? Does this illness know no bounds of Horror and deprivation? Then I started to think what I did yesterday and the day before, "NOTHING" "ABSOLUTELY NOTHING " came to mind but as I asked Elaine what we did and as she told me a little bit of recognition came back and I remembered a few things.

Have I been too wrapped up in everything these last few weeks to notice my decline? Is it a blessing for me not to remember or just a constant curse for my family and friends? Is this the start of my decline? I can't be the only one with a diagnosis who feels or has felt this way but how many have had the confidence to talk about it? How many people want to or wanted to talk about these worries, especially those that were on their own or had very little support?

This is why we MUST!!! Make Dementia a topic to be spoken about and debated about in the open! Not behind closed doors!! And certainly not without involving those of us who actually have this awful disease!! We have a voice as well!! Who better to tell it "AS IT IS" than us and not what some who "THINK" what it is. We have to involve all Carers" from all walks of life as their "up close and personal" experience is absolutely invaluable, including families' and loved ones who have all had their own journeys and stories to tell. Please join me on my journey to make the Stigma of Dementia a thing of the past. If I am in Decline I promise you all I will not go down without a fight!!

Never A Dull Moment

Well, as you have probably guessed there is never a dull moment in our lives!! LOL, still, there are times I do long for a bit of peace and quiet and a day without some sort of trauma!!LOL But, with Alzheimer's alone comes many things, from my mind drifting off here and there during the day to totally switching off at times. Lately I have been experiencing some very strange episodes which I can only explain as being in two places at once. Now I know most of my friends will say that I have had a lot to deal with over the last couple of months or so and with my CT scan fast approaching I must admit there have been times I have felt totally desolate and so down in the mouth but this is quite different to what I have been through before. I have found myself thinking about a subject, usually from years ago, or it can be a piece of music from days gone by, and I feel as if I am being transported back to that time in my life and I am experiencing the same thing all over again!! I can't really explain it as a dream state as I am fully conscious; I am physically in the "NOW" but mentally in the past. It's happened a few times now and the only way I can try to explain it is it's like being transported back in time, yet, still knowing somewhere deep inside my brain that I shouldn't be there. I hope this is making sense. It's like living in two worlds and sometimes the world I am in is not very nice and I find myself shouting out loud as if I have Tourrettes!!

The vocal part of it has, thankfully, only happened a couple of times but the mind wandering seems to be more frequent these days. Is it a worrying sign that I could be getting worse? Or is it just the stress I have been under lately? Sadly I think it's the first option but, (and I think you know what's coming next!!LOL) as I always say, whatever the future holds, whatever the results are next week, and whatever I have to face, I am happy and content that I will not be facing this uncertain future alone. With the family and fantastic friends I have I am sure to overcome whatever is thrown at me.

My Journey`s End

Hiya, three years ago when I was first diagnosed with Early onset Alzheimer's I wrote my first ever story about it and decided to share it with the world!. As most of you know I called it "Me and My Alzheimer's" and a book soon followed. That was three years ago and looking back I think I was very naive at the time. I stated that I was on a "Journey" with Alzheimer's" and treated it accordingly. After the recent events of the last week or so I now realise this is not the case and will never will be from now on!! Being on a "Journey "with this awful disease sounds like I am sharing a coach ride to Blackpool for the weekend with it!! It sounds like we have both happily jumped on a National Express Coach together and decided to tour the Highlands of Scotland!!! I now realise this is not the case!!! I am not "On a Journey" with this B****Y thing, I am at WAR with it!! And whichever way I, or other people wrap it up, I am "FIGHTING FOR MY LIFE HERE" and this is exactly what I intend to do!! Maybe some will say "Oh well it's just probably the time of year" or It's been hard year" and both are very true!! But the fact is I know myself and I know my condition has deteriorated. I could write another two/three pages stating how, but I won't, it's bad enough having it, without moaning about it!!LOL LOL As you all know it's not in my Gene`s to whinge about it, in this house we just get on with it, thankfully.

So, where do I go from here??? Well, a trip to my wonderful consultants would be a good start just to see if there is any way of maybe upping the dosage of "Ebixa" (Memantine/Namenda) or even combining two different Alzheimer's medications (Answers on a post card please Ha Ha) Who knows, the new year might even bring a breakthrough cure, it's what we are all hoping for so why not??Until then my friends, I promise you this, I will as long as humanely possible, I will keep up the awareness raising and trying to change things for the better, and besides, I WONT let Alzheimer`s Catch up with me just yet I HAVE TOO MUCH TOO DO!!

One Of Those Days

Have you ever had one of those days?

When you should have stayed in bed,

When you put shampoo on your toothbrush,

Instead of on your head,

When your false teeth just don't fit,

And they don't feel as if they`re yours,

And all you want to do all day,

Is walk through different doors,

When your jumpers on inside out,

And stuck above your head,

When nobody can find you,

As your sitting in your shed,

This is what dementia does,

To me and many others,

But we are in a special group,

My sisters and my brothers,

Some may face this daily,

But with head held high,

As we end our day with a smile,

And not a fearful cry

Out Of Sight Out Of Mind

How many times do we hear that in our life and how many different scenario`s can it apply to? I can certainly think of one especially when the word "Dementia" is mentioned in some circles. But this is my personal take on it and is something that happened the other day. My own "Out of sight, out of mind feeling took on a brand new meaning to me as I went out with (my Angel) Elaine for some lunch. If you recall a few days ago it was an absolute washout regarding the weather and torrential rain was coming down in Torquay. We have never been the "Staying in" kind so Elaine decided we should treat ourselves to some lunch at a nearby pub. As we arrived there was hardly anywhere to park so Elaine dropped me off at the front and hunted for somewhere to park. This started a chain of events that were very worrying for me at the time and a completely new experience for me. I stood inside the foyer for what seemed like an age and I become more and more aware of people looking at me, or so i thought? I have never been paranoid and always say that people have to find me as I am, but this was different. As I scanned the outside for Elaine I saw her face smiling at me and she was waving to me. I was so relieved but tried not to show it but without much success. We found a table, ordered our lunch and had a small intimate chat about how I was feeling. The lunch was lovely and it was onward and upward to M+S to have a look at the new upstairs they have just built. But that wasn't the end of it. Elaine once again dropped me off whilst she parked, at my insistence I might add, and there I stood. Within minutes self doubt started to creep into my mind and as time went on I stated to physically panic. The thoughts flying around in my head were of

"How did I get here? " Did I imagine Elaine bringing me here?" "Where am I?" and Am I dreaming all this? As Elaine is not here I must be!! I stood rooted to the spot not even moving for people who were trying to get past which must have seemed very unusual to say the least. Time seemed to tick away so so slowly and almost stood still in my mind.

I could feel a scream welling up inside me of sheer panic and lack of understanding, not only of the feeling of loneliness and helplessness but of realising that this was yet another stage of this awful terrible disease trying to drag me down into its depths of despair. Just then as I looked up I saw Elaine hurrying through the door at some speed, somehow realising my plight from afar and taking a hold of my arm and giving me a great big hug. I didn't know whether to laugh, cry or just shout out at the sheer relief I felt at that moment and we must have looked like two lovers who had not seen each other for a long time. But I didn't care, Elaine was there, I hadn't imagined it all, and I knew then, all would be ok. All this happened just because there was nowhere to park because of the weather, it was nobody`s fault, but it just shows you how something so seemingly innocent can affect the thinking of someone like me who has Dementia. Is this disease "Out Of Sight out of Mind" for some people? Do they deny the existence of dementia and just put it down to old age?

Try walking in my shoes for a while!!

To all those affected by this terrible disease you will know only too well the way this disease destroys you and your loved ones bit by bit and painfully slowly and how it affects your lives on a day to day basis. Hopefully this will go some way to describing what it's like and helps more people understand this God awful disease.

OUT OF THE MOUTH`S OF BABE`S

Hiya all, just had to tell you all this. As we arrived at the holiday camp Elaine got very busy putting things away in the holiday home (Caravan) whilst I was in the front room with my grandchildren, Brionie aged 12yrs and Colby aged 9yrs when Colby Aged nine asked a question, the conversation went something like this: "Grandad, what's wrong with you??" "He`s got Alzheimer's" replied Brionie, What's Alzheimer`s asked Colby?" "Well, "said Brionie, it's when you start to forget things and remember things isn't it Grandad? "Yes it is darling" I replied whilst looking at Colby with interest as I knew this question would be coming very soon from him". RUBBISH!!!!! Colby shouted at Brionie as if I wasn't there, Grandad remembers tons of stuff about when he was younger and teaches us all sorts of things about growing up and stuff!!! How can you say he forgets things? He told us lots of things coming here in the car and every time I ask him something and he answers it for me, I always say "How do you know that Grandad? And he (me) always says "I`m your grandad, it's my job to know!!LOL LOL"

But its true isn't it grandad, that's what Alzheimer's is, isn`t it?? (Believe it or not she has read my book!!)

So the next ten minutes I had to explain to a very confused nine year old who loves his grandad very much that now and again I might just forget a few things in the future and might not know as many answers as I usually do. He was visibly crestfallen and looking a little jaded. Ads Their Nana (Elaine) shouted them Colby turned round to me and asked "Grandad, who was the first man on the moon?" Neil Armstrong!! I answered quickly!! SEE!! Shouted Colby to his big sister, I told you he was only joking as usual!!LOL So maybe I will wait until he is a bit older before I try explain it to him again, in the meantime who am I to destroy his dream, I am sure I can muddle through a little bit longer, and by then they may have a cure, and the thought of his Grandad forgetting anything will be soon forgotten by him....................................Hopefully

Past Times

I look through eyes that are so old,

I walk on feet that feel so cold,

Was it all that long ago?

When I was 21 and in the know, My

mind wanders way back when, We

ran though fields, down the glen,

Now my mind, is so still,

Memories faded, body ill,

Names and face`s fade away,

Memory playing tricks all day,

I am just an empty shell,

Existing through this living hell,

Words I once held so dear

Won't come out, without the fear,

Of making sense of what I say, To

live like this from day to day

Sometimes I want to say goodbye,

Just lay my weary head and sigh,

To say goodnight to one and all,

And Wait to hear my Gods call,

But until then, I have no choice,

To try and speak through silent voice,

I promise to try and do my best,

Until the day I come to rest

Living Day To Day

I went to a meeting yesterday of the Torbay Dementia Leadership Group of which I am lucky enough to be Chairperson of. One of the things we discussed was how important it is for an early diagnosis. We all more or less agreed that there was some sort of downfall on the local Doctors Part (but not all of them) as some of them still see Dementia as nothing more than an aging problem and old age and dementia comes hand in hand!! (Is this the same in the USA PLEASE??) This is one part of the fight to raise awareness that must be addressed. I personally can't express how IMPORTANT an early diagnosis is!!! And why wouldn't you want to know?? I can fully understand that some people don't want to and I respect their decision but it still baffles me as to why. The way I look at it is "If you were going into Battle, wouldn't you want to know all about your enemy? Their strengths, their weaknesses ECT??" The more you are informed, the more you learn how to deal with it and how to deal with others when the awkward questions come along, and make no mistake, they will!!! On a more personal note the time I have spent with my family these last three years have been amongst the best of my life and I wouldn't have wanted to miss a single moment of them. There has been many happy times and also many tears along the way in the three years I have been diagnosed and whilst I know the "Clock is Ticking" it doesn't stop me trying to carry on enjoying every minute of it. Some people have asked me if I had one wish what would it be, and the answer is always the same "A CURE" nothing more nothing less. Money and material thing mean absolutely nothing if you haven't got your health. I have sat and cried a million tears both alone (Dementia sufferers are very good at hiding things) and with my family but at the end of the day we have to carry on!! Life just doesn't stop because you have a diagnosis!!! The easiest thing in the world is to give up!!! What's the old saying? "It's better to die as a Lion than a Lamb" Wise words indeed and even for those of us who don't feel like fighting it, then those of us that do, must be there for them to share our strength and help and support them.

Some people don't have the same strength as others do so we must be there for each and every one of them in this fight we call life. As for me and my family, we take it day by day and try to enjoy every moment of it.

Losing My Independence

I love my life!! I know that may sound strange from someone who has heart troubles and a diagnosis of early onset Alzheimer's, but life in general is great because of my family and friends, well, all apart from Wednesdays that is!! Let me explain. Just before Christmas it was agreed that to give my "Angel" Elaine a very well earned rest I would have a community support worker to come and "Sit" with me for a couple of hours once a week (on a Wednesday) whilst Elaine can go and spoil herself a little and do things without having to keep an eye on me all the time. My new "friend" came round a couple of times and is due round again this week after the Christmas break. As I awake every Wednesday I feel as if I have lost yet another little piece of my independence which will never be brought back. I am in such turmoil! On the one hand there isn't anything I would not do for "My Angel" Elaine as she has done more for me that I, or you, could ever imagine, BUT!!!! Having to have someone to come and "SIT" with me for two hours is something I am having a real problem with. Please don't get me wrong, this guy is a nice enough bloke and is quite easy to talk to but the thought of having to be looked after by a complete stranger horrifies me. I look in Elaine's eyes sometimes and I see how tired she is, my heart sinks and the feeling of guilt is overwhelming!! It hurts me so much that I am putting my soul mate through this each and every day. I am sure others in my position must think the same but just don't always say so. It's a feeling that is so hard to explain, all I want to do is make things easier for her and her future (my fate is sealed unless they find a cure, of that I am certain, and I have come to terms with that) so by giving her time to "Chill out" for the want of a better word and helping her to relax more is a fantastic thing!! Again BUT???? Whilst this is happening I feel as if a little more of my independence is slipping away bit by bit and being the fighter that I am, my whole body/mind and being is resisting it!! It has come to the point now where I can get very low on these days, as well as frustrated and even annoyed. My whole mood changes as the time approaches and I start to go inward and withdraw into myself so the conversation is practically NIL when my "Friend" arrives.

Am I being selfish?? I really don't want to be and I really don't know if the answer is yes, or no! Truth be told, since my heart troubles started Elaine has been my full time carer now for the last eight/nine years and I have not even been out through the door on my own in all that time purely for my own safety, and since the diagnosis of AD I have no road sense whatsoever and it would now be fatal for me to try and cross a road on my own.

The thing I am also struggling with is the news that this is going to be a PERMENANT arrangement!! This is what is totally throwing me at the moment; I think it's the sheer enormity of FOREVER!!! That frightens me to death!! Once again I start to think "Is this the start of   Denial of my illness beginning to creep in? Am I eventually going to be heard saying "There is nothing wrong with me because I can't remember being diagnosed?? Can anybody imagine what's going through my head at the moment? And how many people before me have gone through this exact same thing and had these exact same feelings?? I wonder how many people have spoken about this and discussed the implications of this happening. Nobody ever tells you this when you are first diagnosed!! Nobody ever says "there might come a time when even though you are very aware what is going on in the world, apart from a few things you forget, you will have to sit opposite a complete stranger in your own house and talk about nothing!! Such is the devastation of DEMENTIA!! This is how it feels when you feel like bits of your independence is being chipped away slowly and clinically. Without a doubt this is one of the worst kinds of illnesses, it robs you of so many things, it hurts everybody around you without a fleeting care and causes rifts, arguments and tensions beyond belief. Elaine is my soul mate, my best friend and everything I have ever wanted, I can count on one hand the times we have had a big falling out, and I feel so bad about her not having time to herself, but the feeling of insecurity and loneliness when she is not here is a soul destroying thing and I wouldn't wish it on anybody!!

The Answer? I haven't got one at the moment I'm afraid, I only wish I had. It might only seem a couple of hours a week to some, and I'm sure it feels like that for my darling Elaine as well!!

But it feels like a lifetime to me and to be perfectly honest about it I am having a really hard time at the moment dealing with it. I am sorry this is not my usual upbeat post but I just want to share with you some of the "Hidden" feelings we have to go through and deal with regarding this awful illness.

Maybe I will get used to it? Or maybe as I said, I may just forget what my "Friend" is coming for and just put up with it? Who knows?

Memories Of Music

Music plays such a big part in my life. If I am in the kitchen, The radio`s on, if we are eating a meal, the CD`s are on and even in the bathroom the radio plays away as I wash and shave. Because of my night terrors (which can keep half the street up!! LOL) I now go to bed about an hour before my wife and listen to my local radio station through my headphones on my walkman and have found that because of this my night terrors have almost diminished into nothing but normal nightmares. Who knows why? But if it works for me then it gives everybody else including my long suffering "Angel" Elaine some much needed sleep!! Last night whilst listening to the radio it played an hour of the sixties and a number one from 1967 called "When you Going to San Francisco" Suddenly I was transported back to being 10 years old again. I felt the same nervousness as I did way back then about leaving primary school and going on to big school. As I closed my eyes I imagined being sat there on a cushion in front of the telly at mum and dad's with the fire roaring at my back. At the side of me were two wall cupboards where mum used to keep all her shoe polishes and dads tools were in there as well. I could actually smell the Cherry Blossom polish wafting up my nose like a smell of a long gone age. On the television was wrestling from the Wryton Stadium with Mick Mc Manus and the Royal Brothers. I was ten again and loved every minute of it!!! Before I knew it I had opened my eyes and I was back in my bed in Torquay (With Alzheimer's) and the reality of everything that is going on hit home once again!!

BUT!!! And as you know, there is usually a BUT with me, this got me thinking???? There are some great groups starting up in this country regarding Dementia and particularly in the south west of England where I live called "Singing for the Brain" Amongst people with Dementia this has proved to be a great success in helping people who have been withdrawn to come out of their shell a little more and not only to join in the singing but remembering the song without looking at the words!

These are great strides towards helping people who suffer from this awful disease to learn how to socialise again and get a little bit of their memories back as well as a little independence. I am honoured that I have been asked to speak as guest speaker on the recruitment drives to hopefully find volunteers all over the south west of England to set up these "Singing for the Brain" groups and hopefully help them on their way to being successful. Adding to this I wondered if it would be a good idea not only to play songs from "Long Ago" to a loved one or a client, but also music from five or ten years ago, as sometimes memories from long ago are the last to go and as I know from personal experience these are easy to remember, it's the last few years/months that I have trouble with. A conversation could be held with loved ones and relatives to find out if the person with dementia enjoyed a particular concert just before being diagnosed, or what was their favourite music which they have forgotten? This could then be played to see if there is a reaction or a memory stirred from within? I have always thought that music plays a much bigger part in our lives than we realise so to play music from down the years and not just from years ago could be so beneficial. I suppose the million dollar question is "Does it help me?" And my answer is a resounding YES!!!! So if it works for me, it might just work for others.

I hope you don't mind me sharing this with you as hopefully I have helped to maybe, in my own humble way, to stir a few memories amongst people with this awful disease, and if not, I would love to bet they enjoyed the music anyway so what harm can it do???LOL LOL

My Grandson!!!

(I would just like to explain that I recently appeared on television and was raising awareness for the drug Ebixa which has stalled my onset of Alzheimer's, this was my grandsons take on it !!)

"How old are you Grandad?" "53yrs old came my reply"

WOW!! That's really old isn't it?

This is how the conversation started with my five year old grandson Mac, as we sat on my reclining (almost fully reclined just the way we like it loll) chair watching Horrid Henry; He was snuggled into my shoulder so far he was almost coming out the other side. These are times I cherish and will (Hopefully) keep with me forever. I tried to explain to him that 53yrs old isn't really that old but the look in his eyes said he was having none of it loll !! He carried on "I saw you on television the other day, did you see me waving to you?" I explained I couldn't see him but I gave him a great big squeeze for doing so and kissed his cheek. Could I just explain at this point that Mac is only five years old but has quite clearly "BEEN HERE BEFORE!! LOL and has the wit and the wisdom of a 30yr old. "I told my teacher that you had been on television but I told him I was a bit worried about you" he said with that innocent look in his eyes, yet, in the pit of my stomach I knew something was brewing!!

"What do you mean??" was my tentative reply.

"Well" he said taking a big breath, when I saw you on telly they said you were on DRUGS!!!! But I told my teacher that wasn't true as only bad people took drugs!!

There was an ALMIGHTY COUGH!! As Elaine almost choked on her coffee and chaos ensued. My eight year old grandson was in a fit of giggles as the thought of his dear old grandad on drugs must have hit a funny bone!!

The five year old sat in the knave of my arm was sat there looking bemused at all the fuss and I couldn't believe what I had just heard!!LOL LOL In my eighteen years or so as a grandad (You can work the maths out loll) I have never ever been as stuck as to what to say in my defence!! I was wild-eyed and open mouthed. So, let's get this straight I said very nervously, "You told all your teachers that I was on telly but the telly said I was taking drugs but you said it wasn't true because I'm your grandad and I wouldn't do something like that? "YES" he said quite proudly. Lost for words is SUCH an understatement at this point and I must have looked as though I was in a mime act as my mouth was moving but no sound was coming out!! I looked across at Elaine in sheer panic and mouthed the word HELP!!! Elaine, as cool as ever, asked Mac to join her on the settee, so he did a swap with his older brother who was still in fits of laughter at what hit little brother had just come out with. With Mac sitting still and listening to his Nana as if his life depended on it (you can tell who the soft one is in this house, nannies defiantly the boss LOL) she had to explain that there are good drugs and bad drugs and the good drugs are only taken by good people who get them from a Doctor on prescription and not naughty people!! What a Genius my Elaine is!! Never in a million years would I have thought of that!! How much of this he actually understood we really don't know but sanity was resumed, well for ten minutes anyway. This just shows how this awful illness of Dementia affects families in more ways that you could ever dream of. Actually having to have such a conversation like this with two of my grandsons just shows you how important it is to find a cure. Children and adults are put in this position every day and shouldn't be. Children especially, they are the innocents and our future. They should be allowed to have their childhood without these worries. Still, I suppose looking back now it was kind of funny!!!LOL. Will I let them watch a future TV appearance?

I DONT THINK SO!!! I haven't been with Elaine to pick them up from school since, I wonder why??? LOL

My Words For You

Sitting quietly, not really there,

All seeing eyes, yet vacant stare

Mouth that moves, but does not speak

Words are whispered, from one so weak,

Future fading in failing mind,

Sudden release would be so kind,

Confusion reigns all around,

Screaming out, yet not a sound,

Trapped inside a mind of Pain,

Feeling nothing left to gain,

Please hear my voice, I'm still here,

With shaking hands and falling tears,

Remember me as I do you,

Remember all the good times too,

From deep inside please know this,

I cherish your embrace and kiss,

So until that day, when we part,

Always know you have my heart

Night Sky Of Hope

Hiya, where we live in Torquay we are quite fortunate as in we live in a nice flat in an old Victorian house. Because of this we have floor to ceiling windows in our front room so the views are quite clear. At night time this especially so and last night I found myself staring at the night sky. Its complete blackness and enormity made me feel very humble and the more I thought about it the more I thought about how we look at dementia. The darkness and blackness descends without warning, with no sound, omitting most of the brightness of the day. It creeps up on us daily and there are no warning signs, no alarm bells or "Symptoms" as such, in the early stages of the night times and before you know it, it's completely dark!! Does this sound familiar?? Mmm, very familiar to me, BUT!! (And as you know there is always a BUT with me LOL) when you look into this sheer darkness what also can you see?? What I saw last night was the shiniest star I have ever seen, maybe I am noticing more these days, some say you do when you're really ill, but through all that darkness and density was this star, shining and twinkling in the depth of blackness like I had never seen before. Against all the odds, there it was, shining a light that started millions of years ago but still living on pulsating in the night sky. Then, as I looked around, there was another, and another, and another!!!!! My heart skipped a beat and I felt as if I was an excited child all over again, WHY??? Because in my mind all these wonderful shining stars were rays of hope!! Each and every one of them held the hope and prayers of everybody who is touched by this awful illness, every single one of them was somebody who had the hope and faith that one day a cure would be found, and this was the universes way of saying HOLD ON!! A Cure is coming and coming soon!! Every star that shines so bright is the light of belief that we all hold on to so dear. So the next time you take a look up, and stare at the wonderment of the universe, just give thanks, that all the lights you see will be shining so much brighter in the very near future.

(Since writing this on Jan 3rd 2011 A UK and World Dementia Awareness Day were created and it happens on September 17th every year. At the time of writing this it's just gone GLOBAL and we have over 11,000 pledges on the Face book causes Page "Help set Up A Uk Dementia Awareness Day ")

As The World Turns

As the world turns slowly round each day, life goes on. Everyday a new challenge is thrown up at us to adapt to and overcome. As we all know for some, one of those challenges is Alzheimer's. So what can we do to "adapt and overcome" as I always say? You will probably know by now that I passionately feel that Awareness is the key and will one day rid this awful disease of the terrible stigma that's attached to it!! But what I want to talk about today from a personal experience is "Early Diagnosis" I think that the key, not only to acceptance of this disease but the betterment and quality of life is an early diagnosis!! I was diagnosed at 50yrs old, went steadily downhill for a few months until I was given the drug Ebixa, and I can honestly say I have just spent the most wonderful 18 months with my incredible family and friends!! I shudder to think that I could have missed out on all this if I hadn't been diagnosed or been misdiagnosed because I am "so young" for such a disease!!!

To make sure this happens many things have to be put in place and these things unfortunately take time. From making sure GP's Dr,s, Consultants and all professional people don't dismiss it as behavioural problems instead of a Dementia, to family being open and honest about what they are seeing happening to a loved one or friend. All these things need to be put in place to make sure the WORLD WAKES UP TO DEMENTIA!!! Here come the "IFS" but just think about this for a moment. IF I hadn't been diagnosed, IF I hadn't seen a consultant, IF I hadn't been prescribed the drugs I have been described I would have by now LOST everything I hold so precious, dear and close to me. I would have lost moments that I now cherish and will for too for the rest of my life. And here comes the big "IF" "IF "I myself had DENIED having the disease and refused treatment I am fully convinced that the disease would have taken over my brain, and it would certainly be too late now to be treated!!!! That's how serious it is, we are dealing with "LIFE OR DEATH" here, whichever way you want to wrap it up, that's a fact!!!

So what can WE do?? The word I will always use and come back to is EDUCATE PEOPLE by RAISING AWARENESS!! YES ITS THAT SIMPLE!! I was told the other day that no matter what comes or goes in September I have still raised awareness to over 9,000 people up to now and still counting!!! Can you imagine the good we could do if we all do just half of that!!!

I wish you all so much happiness my friends and always remember

WHERE THERE IS LIFE, THERE IS HOPE!!!

Burgers Children And Alzheimer`s

Hello my friends just thought I would tell you about our visit to a well known burger bar (BK) with two of my grandsons, Colby aged 9 and McKenzie aged 6 but thinks he is 50yrs!! Old I haven't been with Elaine picking them up over the winter months because of my illnesses and the weather, but today I ventured out because I had promised to take them for a burger and it was blue sky all the way!! If ever I wanted another reason to fight with all my might against this awful disease dementia, the look in my grandson's eyes as they saw me waiting for them with their Nan (Elaine) was another "MESSAGE TO BRAIN" never, ever to give up the fight. Their smiles lit up the play ground and they both held onto me like their life's depended on it!!LOL You would never imagine we had only seen each other two days earlier!! So off to the burger bar we went in the car and within seconds the questions were coming thick and fast!! WHY? WHAT? WHEN? And they all had the word "GRANDAD" in front of them; I was convinced they had forgotten their Nan's name!! LOL Well as you can imagine, I have trouble at the best of times listening at normal speed but always wanting to please, I tried my best to fire the best answers I could back at them, and in turn where possible LOL

I didn't do too badly for the first ten minutes; I was quite pleased with myself!!HaHaHa, but it went a little downhill from there as I was answering the totally wrong questions and eventually talking about something completely different!!! But do you know something? I didn't care, and you know why? Because I was having the best time of my life and it carried on in the Burger bar as well!! Messing about, rocking with laughter, being very loud and boisterous. For those sixty minutes or so the worry of this fatal disease creeping up on me was totally vanquished!! All was well with the world and nothing mattered apart from the loved ones I was with at the time!! I know sometimes i write about how hard it is and how and far this awful road this illness can take you, but sometimes, just sometimes, things like this happen and it just makes life and the fight all WORTHWHILE!!!

This is one of these times and I just couldn't wait to get home and share it with you my dear friends, I shall sleep the sleep of the peaceful tonight, that's if I ever stop giggling at the sight of my cheeky grandsons faces!!!

Beating Heart

Beating heart, don't be still

Just because, I am ill, Tired

eyes, weary legs,

Find a cure, my heart begs,

Very tired of this venture, In

this fight with Dementia,

So much pain, so much sorrow,

Praying for a new tomorrow,

Until that day, a cure is found,

Let our hopes and dreams abound

So beating heart, don't be still,

Just because I am ill

Autumns On Its Way

As autumn leaves start to fall, and winters on its way,

There`s a chill, in the air, with the shorter days,

The soups and stews all arrive, and start to smell so good,

Like meeting good old friends again, it's always in your blood,

The heating gets turned on, from its summer rest,

If you have old fashioned coal, the hearth it looks its best,

A roaring fire is what I miss, with ashes, mess and all,

With flames a golden yellow, shooting up so tall,

Your breath appears from your mouth, like the Papal smoke,

And forgetting to put your woollies on, really is no joke,

These bones of mine feel it now, as I am growing old,

I seem to shiver more these days, as I feel the cold,

So up and closer I will move, towards my roaring fire,

And put another layer on so I won't feel so dire

Anguished Cries

Anguished cries through the night,

Alzheimer's holds my dreams so tight

Invading every single scene,

Always knowing where I've been,

Thrashing legs, flaying arms,

My "Angel" Elaine, staying calm,

Gently wakes me from my hell,

Saving me from his deathly Knell,

Another night has been survived,

Whatever next will he contrive?

But I will be ready, no matter what,

He has planned, because I have got,

My "Angel" here next to me,

So my defeat, he will never see

CHANGING TIME`S

Well!! It's been quite a week!! Travelling to Bournemouth for the Dementia Congress and one thing and another! I am sure I am much better when I'm kept busy, but just before we set off on our travels I had time to think about what is happening around me and how I feel I am changing, and make no mistake, I am changing within myself, which is confusing in itself, let alone for anybody else to understand but I will give it a try. You know when sometimes you just feel out of sorts and just feel like you are coming down with something? Well, it's like that but on a more personnel level. I blurted out something two days ago which not only came as a surprise to me but my whole family who were there at the time and I will not repeat it as it wasn't very nice!! I find myself wandering in my mind more often, and I keep remembering things that happened what only seemed like yesterday but in reality it was many years ago. I am more distracted now than I was and find it hard to concentrate at anything without a huge effort being made. Some will say we have had a lot on lately with our daughter going away and the conference but I think this is different. I just don't feel as if I am myself anymore!!

I know this is probably hard to understand but it's like my personality is ebbing away slowly and being replaced with a feeling of emptiness and loneliness which as you know is not like me. My sleeping pattern is not the same and my nighttimes are as bad as ever, if not worse. I seem to drift through the day some days and can't even remember where or what I have done that morning. This is not all of the time, just some days, just drifting and never really connecting. But when my days are of some clarity I see the world in my own "Happie Chappie Way" and just wonder at the marvels of life around me and all its glory. I still can't quite believe that someone like me (just a boy from Lancashire) managed to make a huge company like BUPA re- write their booklet on Dementia care and make (Hopefully) such a difference to all the people under 65 who are unfortunate enough to have this awful disease.

Mine was just one voice, and the one thing that keeps my spirits up is if just little old me can manage something like this, can you just imagine what we can achieve if we all raise our voices high and TOGETHER AS ONE!!!!

I have always lived by the saying

"If you always do, what you have always done,

You will always get what you have always got!!

And I truly believe that we can all make such a difference if we try.

When I saw my specialist last week who also gets my e mails HA HA, she said that she had noticed a downturn in my mailings and also when we spoke there was a definite downturn in my health regarding the dementia so at the moment I am not too sure how I am going to feel in the coming months and as you know I always live for the day, but I promise you all this from the bottom of my heart, no matter how things work out in the near future I will always be flying the flag for Dementia sufferers young and old and will continue to do so for as long as both Physically and mentally possible.

I will never give up the fight! And let's hope this is just a BLIP!!LOL LOL

Children's Questions And An Uncertain Future

Yesterday was spent with my two youngest grandsons and my eleven year old granddaughter who is growing up fast!! She has just moved to secondary school and becoming more curious by the day. During the day the conversation turned to what she wanted to do in the future, her hopes and dreams. We are a very close family and talking about these things comes easy, but, trying to keep a smile on my face as she talks about the next few years was hard to do. She asked about future Christmas`s and her growing into a teenager and hopefully becoming a vet but there is time yet to change her mind (as she quickly reminded me) As many of you know I am not usually stuck for words LOL and especially where my grandchildren are concerned but I must admit I struggled a little yesterday and with the emotional attachment that goes with it, it was a trying time. The look in her eyes of expectation and hope for the future was absolutely wonderful to see and all my hopes and love are invested in her. But, what about the uncertainty of my future and how do I keep up the facade? It`s certainly a tough one. As we said goodbye to them yesterday I gave my granddaughter a big special hug and thought about what was to come. How do I answer her questions in future? How do I say with confidence and honesty that I will always be there for her as I have always been since she was born? And how do I not lie to her when she says "Promise me Grandad?"

As an Alzheimer's sufferer when I was first told of this illness nobody but nobody can prepare you for this kind of emotional turmoil. There are no rules or regulations to this awful disease apart from the certainty of the outcome unless they find a cure! Nobody says "Hey!! I know of a book that tells you what to do and how to deal with things like this! Yes there are a few booklets to advise on how to answer any awkward questions from children but the reality of it is when those questions are asked its life changing and so emotional you are never really prepared for it.

My love for my family and children is unquestionable and undying and I will always believe it will be, but at times like this it completely throws you no matter how hard you try to say it doesn't and the feeling of emptiness and helplessness can completely consume you and throw you into a pit of despair. These are the feelings and things people never tell you about or talk about, these are some of life's hardest lessons to learn when you are an Alzheimer's sufferer. I can deal with the "I am going to die "part as I have had such a wonderful life and couldn't have wished for a more loving and supportive family. I can deal with "I have so much to do yet" as I have done so much, seen so much and been as lucky as any man can be through life, but what I have trouble dealing with is the fact that chances are I will NOT see my children's dreams become a reality and be a part of them, and I will NOT see the look on their eyes as they achieve all they want to in life.

Alzheimer's wants to take all this away from me, but I promise you as I have promised myself, NOT IF I HAVE ANYTHING TO DO WITH IT!!!!

"Where There is life There Is Always Hope"

Dark Day

And to think yesterday started out so well. We were up and out early doing some last minute shopping, well truth be told, we have never been so disorganised as this year because we have been so busy, so I suppose we were just catching up!! In all the excitement I had forgotten that I had to have a blood test at 1-20 pm yesterday afternoon with a new nurse at the surgery. I will at this point just say that for those of you who don't know, I have a huge phobia of needles!! s the time neared I found myself getting more and more anxious and sitting in the waiting room felt like I was under sentence of death!! When it was my turn the nurse came out to greet us (As is common practice in our Drs, no Buzzers saying "NEXT" for us thank you. After the usual pleasantries Elaine explained that I had Alzheimer's and a huge fear of needles I advised the nurse that she would only get one shot at this blood taking. She replied" I can't guarantee that", to which I quickly replied "no, BUT I CAN!!LOL LOL"

Well as much as "My Angel "being there and as much as she tried to calm me nothing worked and as soon as metal contacted skin that was it!!! I screamed as it hurt so much and as I realised the nurse hadn't hit a vein first time, things just went from bad to worse!! I sat there in utter disbelief that something had hurt so much and yet I still hadn't had the blood taken!! The next ten minutes were just a repeat of the same question "Please lie down and have it done again? But no matter how much Elaine and the nurse tried to persuade me I wasn't budging. Eventually frustration/Alzheimer's/temper? I don't know but I just got up and stormed out, shirt hanging out and my hands twirling everywhere to get it back on.

Elaine came after me and it was decided the best thing was to leave it for then and Elaine drove me two miles from the Drs, into the countryside and for a coffee at a local organic farm.

As I sat there still shaking I couldn't believe I had behaved so rudely but as Elaine sat down with me, smiled and said "don't worry all will be ok" I started to calm down a little. After a while (and my coffee) Elaine went on to explain that I really had to have this done as the pains I had been having at the side of my head and face could be heart related

(As I have heart failure as you know) I sat and listened as to why I should have it done, and then said my peace. I looked my "Angel" in the eyes, held her hands across the table and said

"Darling, a heart Attack would be a blessed release compared to what I am looking at in the future"

These are words which should never have to be said by any man or lady to their loved ones!!!

These are words that wouldn't NEED to be said if there was a cure for this awful illness.

THESE ARE WORDS THAT ARE SAID BECAUSE OF THIS AWFUL ILLNESS!!

I probably said it a little louder than I had first though as it went so very quiet in the cafe at the farm. But I had said it, and I had hated saying it. It was like the words had come from nowhere and yet wanted to be said for a long time now!! As I looked at my "Angel" I could see the hurt in her eyes and my heart felt as if it had snapped and fallen to the pit of my stomach like a heavy sack of potatoes. The next couple of minutes that passed felt like an hour, then, slowly and surely Elaine looked at me, squeezed my hand and said "I know, and I do understand, but what am I to do? I only want what is best for you. We chatted for the next few minutes and calm reigned again. I think this is the time to say that for all you wonderful carer`s / professionals out there, who do their upmost best without thanks or though for themselves and who give their love, dedication and passion without a second thought, that if this ever happens to them, it is not their fault!!

Sometimes, just sometime`s, the person with dementia will be stubborn just like I was and they will want to get their own way, in my case it was something that needed to be said but only came out at the height of a very bad Anxiety attack!!

Does this mean I will be giving up the fight against Alzheimer's?? NOT ON YOUR NELLY!!!! Does this mean I shall be going back to the Drs for my blood test?? Mmm, will get back to you on that one.

DAY BY DAY

As each hour passes day by day,

Sometimes struggling what to say,

Fog and clouds inside my head,

Cannot speak what should be said,

Frustration reigns and tempers flare

Feel so alone with no one there,

Family friends are all around,

Yet in my head, deafening sounds,

Sounds of loneliness' and despair,

Sometimes all too much too bear,

Tears flow, from my eyes,

Sobbing sounds, anguished cries,

Never felt so alone,

This illness always sets the tone,

But in these depths, of despair,

My "Angel" Elaine is always there,

I`m not lonely for very long,

As we sing our favourite song,

DAY`S OF OUR LIVES

Please don't think it's all doom and gloom,

With this illness of mine,

Most days we are happy

Laughing most the time,

You have to take it day by day,

And not worry about tomorrow,,

It's so easy to get dragged down,

And wallow in your sorrow,

I wake up every morning,

With one thing on my mind,

To survive another day,

Life can be so kind,

So live each day as best you can,

Don't worry about tomorrow,

Because when you're gone forever,

There will be plenty of time for sorrow

Demon Dreams

As I lay me down to sleep,

In my dreams the Demons creep,

Alzheimer's/Dementia will be there,

Causing chaos without a care,

Running wild within my mind,

Screaming shouting, never kind,

Reminding me of days of old,

But yesterday is not so bold, As I

awake with body shaking, Rubbing

eyes, my mind awakening, Trying to

focus, pitch black night, Wide

awake, full of fright,

Beads of sweat run amok,

Whimpering softly, still in shock,

I slowly realise I'm still here,

Wiping away a salty tear,

Again I lay me down to sleep,

And hope my demons cease to creep

Dreaming While awake?

Hiya, i thought i would share my latest experience with you all so hopefully someone can shed some light on it.

Lately, and i know this is going to sound so strange, i have started to dream and shout statements out loud but i am convinced i am totally awake!! When this happens i am always resting in my chair so maybe i am in a dream like state as i do go into Catatonic Trances as i have mentioned before, but i suddenly come round, knowing i have shouted something but have no idea what. On saying that Elaine says she has been talking to me and minutes later i have come out with a statement totally irrelevant to what we were talking about earlier.

Its times like this i am so glad i have had my diagnosis as i wouldn't like to think i was having a breakdown. Now here`s the million dollar question, has anybody else got experience in this kind of thing? And more importantly, is it an indication my condition is worsening??

ECHO`S OF MY PAST

Hiya, as I have mentioned before I seem to be in some sort of transition period at the moment and things are beginning to happen which are so hard to explain, but I promise I will try. I have found myself sort of " Daydreaming more " is the only way I can think of putting it and more and more often every day I seemed to be brought back to reality gently by my (Angel) wife Elaine. In one instance just yesterday Elaine said I was sat there nodding my head as if I were listening to a conversation from someone very close by. Apparently she watched me for a few minutes nodding my head and my eyes going from side to side as if I were understanding every word of it.

This to say the very least is very distressing for Elaine and me as I feel as if I am losing control over what I am able to do and my level of consciousness. One thing I have noticed is my awareness of what's actually going on around me is a lot less than it used to be and lately if I am in town or watching the TV I imagine I can hear voices from people I have known in my past. They are like I have said "Echo`s from my past" sometimes they are more audible than others but never usually make any sense. These I do remember and they shake me up a little to say the least. Sometimes when Elaine or one of my daughters speak to me they sound like my dear mum who only passed away a few months ago as you know. Other times I can be walking through Torquay and I hear my Dad shout, or my best friend Mark, or my brother in law Malc, all whom have been dead for a while now.

Is this the transition I talk about? Is this what happens just before total denial of the illness? My answer is at the moment I don't know, but what I do know is that I have never felt like this before and even though I might not seem any different to the people I know and love, I know myself I that I am.

As well you know people with Dementia are very good at hiding things, but not this one, I just wanted to share with you how I feel at the moment and so hopefully help you understand what we go through from time to time, thank you for listening.

NEVER GIVE UP, WHERE THERE IS LIFE THERE IS HOPE!!

Days Of Hope

Cloudy mind`s, heartfelt cries,

Confusion reigns, tear stained eyes,

Memories fading, yet so aware,

Disappearing without a care,

Aching bones and tired hands,

Time slips like shifting sands,

Waking nightmares every night,

Mouth dry, throat so tight,

Daylight arrives, another day,

With Alzheimer's, never goes away,

Making the best, of my life,

Smiling at my darling wife,

Facing the day with some hope,

It's the only way to cope

Fight Of My Life

I've now come to realise, I'm fighting for my life, And

I would never want, to leave my darling wife, What

about my children, and their children too, Without

their daft old grandad, what are they to do?

I look into my Angels eyes, they sometimes look so sad,

I sometimes hear her crying, over her big lad,

I want to take it all away, removing all the pain,

I just want it to sunshine, and chase away the rain,

To say "it's just not fair", wouldn't sound so right,

There are so many others, with this awful fight,

How do we survive, with Dementia bearing down?

Living day to day, trying not to drown,

Spending every waking moment, with this awful curse,

Knowing every day, it's going to get much worse

Not wanting to look forward, because I can't look back,

Never knowing what will happen, when I go off track

Sometimes it's all too much, trying not to think this way,

And I know it's better, living day by day

So please will you remember me, and remember how I fought,

I hope by my all writings, many I have taught

Getting Ready For The Future

Hiya, as you can imagine these last couple of weeks have been so hectic but during the last two weeks things have been talked about, arranged and things have changed ever so slightly. Beside meetings and lunches there have been a few things going on at home I would like to share with you. As you know we have been on the campaign so to speak to change things for the better, not only for younger early onset but people with Dementia in general. Whilst all this has been going on we have been visited by our CPN (Community Psychiatric nurse), a social worker attached to us and visited us and also a community support worker!!PHEW!! The upshot of it is there are some new sheltered housing flats being opened early next year in Torquay and we have been advised to apply for one. YES!! Again the age limit is 55yrs old (DONT GET ME GOING ON THAT ONE!!LOL) but letters have been written by all our professional friends as well as my consultant explaining that need should be put before age, so here`s hoping.

The thing is, whilst all this paper work and talking about it was being discussed in our front room with the visiting professionals at different times I felt myself being a little excluded from the conversation and you know me, I always want a say in it ! This made me at times think very seriously about my illness and how ill I really am. It seemed to bring it all home to me again what could possibly happen in the future as I get gradually worse and the feeling of sheer helplessness washed over me in waves.

65

It's a tricky one as you can imagine because whilst I want to have peace of mind knowing that "My Angel" will have all the help in place to help her as I get worse, it's a very strange feeling discussing "End of life plans" while able to understand every word of it. Nobody tells you this when you are diagnosed!! Nobody explains that the right thing to do sometimes is talk about your upcoming illness getting so bad that you need to make plans for it! How many more people in my position have had to go through this? And have they had anybody to speak to about it? More importantly how many times has this been discussed in front of a person with dementia without taking their feelings and views into consideration?

(It always ceases to amaze me when you go into homes ECT how many people are dressed without asking what they would like to wear, or are given something to eat without first asking what they would like? Involvement no matter at what stage is so important) But looking back to that couple of weeks I now believe that it was the right thing to do, as I have found I am a little more settled now knowing that the support is in place and ready to help "My Angel" Elaine when the time comes. (Not for years if I have my way!

As I have said before I am a realist and I know, through living it with my father and wonderful grandmother, what the future possibly holds for me if no cure is found, but I do think it's so important to talk about, discuss and try to put people`s mind at ease from very early on.

I am quite prepared to face what will possibly happen to me, so my most important thing for me to concentrate on at the moment is trying to make sure that the journey is also as good as it can be for my wonderful family and of course "My Angel"

Still, food for thought I think if anybody is thinking along the same lines. It has certainly helped us to look forward to a more settled and structured future and I hope by sharing this with you it will help others.

As for the Community Support Worker that's another tale for another day !

Frightened Little Boy

As I tell my tale of Alzheimer`s,

Through smiles and heartfelt joy,

When really, somewhere deep inside

Is just a frightened little boy,

I've faced many things in my life,

Some things too hard to tell,

But Alzheimer`s and all it brings,

Makes my life, a living hell,

Every day a piece of me,

Is lost, forever gone,

It won't give up I know,

Until memories I have none,

So when you see and hear me,

Chatting about my day,

My head rocking back with laughter,

And smiling all the way,

Please spare a thought of what's inside,

Behind the warmth and joy,

Sitting there with head in hands,

Is just a frightened little boy

Hollow Cry`s

Hollow cries from deep inside

Eyes that weep but cannot cry,

Opened mouth and yet no sound,

Familiar voices all around,

Walking round in a dream,

Nothings real, or so it seems,

Waking nights, sleeping days,

Eating meals through foggy haze,

Unfamiliar mirror reflection,

Never right, always correction

All these things and much more,

As Dementia knocks at your door

I`M STILL ME

Hello old friend, sit next to me,

I`m still the man I used to be,

Do you remember way back when?

We played with sticks and built a Den?

And how we ran through cobbled streets,

Drinking Tizer and eating sweets,

The times we had without a care,

Times that I would like to share,

Its yesterday that troubles me,

I can't remember, do you see?

I can remember long ago,

But just last night it isn't so,

But even though my memory`s fading,

Like winter leaves that are shading,

Recent thought`s inside my head,

Now gone forever, almost dead,

But look in my eyes and you will see,

I`m still the man I used to be,

Please old friend, sit next to me

I HATE THIS DISEASE!!

I hate this disease sometimes!! I hate it so much my blood boils and I want to scream!! How dare it invade my brain!! How dare it try to take over my life and take me away from the most precious people in the world , "MY FAMILY " Today we all had such a wonderful day spent with our youngest daughter, her husband and our two youngest grandsons. They emigrate on Sunday so pictures were taken, laughs were heard all over the house and lots of memories, both good and bad but mostly good were re-lived. We filled all our bellies with a corned beef hash (With a crust!!) and bread and butter pudding for our afters. A "Right Good Old Proper Lancashire Send Off" as my wonderful grandmother would have said!! Stories were told and times remembered fondly as the time for them to leave approached. It was quite a quiet goodbye really with not much said but with lots of hugs and kisses and NO TEARS!

Well, not until they had gone!!

As I held Elaine in my arms and listened to her sob very quietly, I stroked her hair and shushed her tears away. Then, after what seemed an age, things were just beginning to settle down when a thought suddenly struck me!! WHAT HAPPENS IF I FORGET THEM ALL? That was it, panic set in and my tears flowed, and with every sob, which started in my feet and ended up coming out of my mouth in violent jerks came a stifled scream. Through the haze I could hear myself saying "WHAT IF I FORGET THEM?" over and over again. Elaine held me tight and said "even if you do they will not forget you"

At that particular moment it did nothing to calm me down and it was only time itself that started to settle me down eventually. I am now three years into my diagnosis and certainly no fool!! Both Elaine,

My Pchycyactric nurse and I have noticed a sharp downturn in my behaviour this last couple of weeks so you can only imagine what was going through my head!! And you wonder why I hate this disease with a vengeance!!

I can only hope and pray that a cure will come soon, very soon, not only for me but for all the others who have to go through this kind of thing and much worse. I am a firm believer that

Where There Is Life There Is Hope"

I WILL NOT GIVE IN TO THIS!!!

Going Too Fast?

Another week over, another week gone,

Not quite sure what happened, not sure what I've done,

I ask my wife and she answers with a smile.

We had a great time and walked mile upon mile,

We saw all the children, took them for a walk,

Listening to them laughing, hearing them talk,

We were one as a family, so close and content,

And all of our children, were heaven sent,

I listened to my wife, and all that we did,

With me on the swings, I'm such a big kid,

So come on you Alzheimer's, you do your worst,

But always remember, my family come first!!

God Bless

Hear My Cries

Voice`s fading, not through age,

Dementia building it`s sound proof cage,

Listening in but nothing out,

Unable to talk but able to shout,

Frustration runs through every bone,

Feeling so empty, always alone,

Hear me cry, silently so,

One day happy, then so low,

I`m still me, deep inside,

Nothing to fear, nothing to hide,

Unable to say what`s on my mind

To those I love, to one so kind,

Hear my cry`s, I'm still here

See my eyes fill with tears,

Until the day we meet again,

And walk among the sunny glen,

Know my heart is always yours,

Until the closing of life`s door`s

I Just Love Spring

I just love spring!! Don't you? All the snowdrops are shimmering in the cold morning light and the Crocuses are just about poking their yellow and purple noses through the soil to have a sniff and see its time to wake up!!

Spring is a time when nature awakens from its winter slumber emerges from the darkness of winter.

(You know where I am going with this don't you??LOL)

It's a time when flowers and trees wake up, stretch and change from the stark emptiness of bare branches and start to bud, just before exploding into leaf. This is nature's time, this is when nature makes a difference and breathes new life into the world and shows everybody that out of darkness can come not only light, but new life, new expectations and new beginnings.

LET'S MAKE THIS SPRING AND YEAR OUR NEW BEGGININGS!!

LET'S BRING DEMENTIA OUT OF THE DARKNESS AND INTO THE LIGHT!!

LET'S BREATHE NEW LIFE INTO THE AWARENESS OF THIS DISEASE!!

AND MOST OF ALL LETS SEE A CURE IN THIS OUR NEW SPRING AND "THE YEAR OF HOPE"

I am fully convinced this is achievable, and with the help of each and every one of you all my dear friends, I know we can do it. We can bring this disease and stigma out of the darkness it's been in for years and years and show people that it's just an illness like any other illness and not one to be hidden or shut away and forgotten about.

I Wish it was September

Hiya, as you know I am not one to be wishing my life away but certain things are happening in my life (health wise) that I don't half wish it was September the 17th and we were all celebrating "Dementia Awareness Day"

With this illness you have highs and lows and dips and troughs health wise. The last couple of days I have felt as if I want to do everything all at once and as quickly as possible. Do I doubt my Mortality? Possibly without realising it? Do I have a feeling deep down that time is running out? All these things run alongside the diagnosis of such a horrendous disease!! But nobody ever tells you this!! Nobody ever tells you about the doubts and fears that creep into your head without warning and takes your world crashing to the floor!!!

It also has other complications as other illness seems to be magnified by this illness and more illness comes along with it. One thing is for sure,

ALZHEIMERS DOESNT COME BY ITSELF!!!

No Sir`eeee!!! So deep down I really wish it was September 17th and the GREAT DAY was in full swing!!!!

But until I will just have to live with the self doubts and the worry as best I can.

I Miss My Mum

It was in June this year, on the 12th day,

When the Angels came and took you away,

You were gone so quick, no time to cry,

Not even time to say goodbye,

I dreamt last night, you were still here,

Sitting next to Dad with nothing to fear,

We were sat having a meal, fish and chips,

With glass in hand, and a smile on your lips,

You looked so young sat next to Dad,

Dining with your eldest lad,

Dad was taken two years before you,

But there you sat, again as two,

Then I awoke and looked around,

And saw nothing but darkness, without a sound,

It was just a dream, a cruel twist,

Of my family who I still miss,

My heart still aches for you dear mum,

From an ever loving son

IN TWO MINDS

I am so angry!!! Not at anybody else, or at myself but at this Dammed Disease!! Whilst I was looking through some computer pics and old postings (something I do regular to remind me hopefully loll) I come to realise I have become two people!! Please stay with me on this as I will try to explain what I feel. I look at pictures of me standing there in front of people with all the confidence in the world trying to raise awareness and forever smiling. Then there is the other me, sitting in my chair, shaking and holding head in hands worrying about the future of my family and what is to become of them.

I have always prided myself as saying "With me what you see is what you get" and I still really believe that, yet the confident me is totally different than the "Worried me" I wonder if that's the difference to having good days and bad? It's sometimes hard to differentiate at times. The confident me is always smiling, always optimistic and forever hoping my life will go on forever. The other me see`s me sat there not saying a word and spiralling into despair about the future. I am already on anti depressants which seem to keep me level, but the difference between the two me`s is astounding!!

Is this all part of the disease? Is it all the up`s and downs a person with dementia goes through? There again I can't remember anybody telling me this would happen? Or did they and I have forgotten?? The frustration wells up inside me and I feel like raging out loud at this disease. How dare you make me feel like this!! How dare you turn me into two different people!!

I AM STILL ME!! AND DONT YOU FORGET IT DEMENTIA DEMON!!!

I am still the same person inside, even though I have my ups and downs, please understand it's only the disease trying to get the better of me, but I won't let it, I am still in here, your friend Norrms, and always will be I WILL NOT LET IT BEAT ME I PROMISE XXX

Is This Denial? Or do I just not remember?

Hiya, as you know we had a great meeting with two very good friends last Friday and it was great to catch up and make plans for the future (ever the optimist loll)

The one thing that did come out of it was my total surprise at some things I (Apparently) do. As we were all chatting I started to listen to Elaine telling one of our friends how I put the Camera in the breadbin and how I can never get the shower right, turning all the dials with no known danger of hot water!! How taking me across the road is like having a three year old with her as I have no idea how to cross a road or have any road sense!! (I must admit I have heard the road sense one before. Not only that I apparently need help with dressing/washing/shaving and getting my socks on!! All news to me!! Well, apart from the socks!! And I think some of the things that I can't do any more were to embarrassing for Elaine to mention!!

I must admit at one stage I was sat there thinking "Who is Elaine talking about??" "I didn`t know we knew somebody else so close who had a diagnosis like me??" Then all of a sudden it hit me like a thunderbolt it was me who Elaine was talking about and I was absolutely GOBSMACKED!! I just sat there and listen to some of the things I had done (I must admit I giggled at some loll) and shook my head whilst pretending I knew what Elaine was talking about!! It wasn't until we got home later that night that we had what I call "A Sit Down Talk" (we all remember them don't we. After explaining to Elaine I couldn't remember half the things she was talking about I began to wonder if a certain amount of denial had started to creep in without me knowing it.

This is what this horrible illness does to you!

This is how it treats you with a total lack of respect!!

This is how it makes me and every other person with this awful illness doubts themselves, their sanity and their lives!!! Make no mistake, as a good friend of mine has said to me, this is the EVIL we have to put up with!!!

Everybody who is touched by this awful disease has to put up with this at one stage or another. Can you imagine being told you have been doing things you have absolutely no memory of and over such a period of time???? Can you imagine how frustrating this is?? And can you imagine what goes through the persons mind as he or she is being told this?? I know what went through my mind but that is unprintable!!LOL So, is this me just being in Denial? Or is it just the nature of the beast we all have to deal with?? To be honest I am not quite sure but one thing I am sure of is

IT WILL NOT BEAT ME!!!! THAT I PROMISE EACH AND EVERY ONE OF YOU!!!

All this will take some time to get used to but get used to it I will, and as long as I have breath in my body I will continue to raise awareness and see a cure to this horrible illness !!!

Just One Question?

It was just one question!! Just one question, as simple as that!! Out of the blue last night my "Angel" Elaine asked me if I missed going out on New Year's Eve. Who would have known that just one question could have evoked such an emotional reaction by me? I sat there and thought about it for a few seconds and answered "yes, of course I do", and this was followed by "And do you know what else I miss?

1 "Getting ready and looking forward to a great night out (Problem being can't fasten my buttons, tie or shoelaces any more)

2 Going to a concert and listening to the groups playing live!! (Problem) Anything loud these days seems to run through me like electricity.

3 Going from pub to pub and having such a laugh with everybody, (Problem) Thanks to the Alzheimer's very low self esteem and confidence.

4 Meeting up at midnight and dancing the New Year in (Problem) too tired to stay up so late.

5 Sitting in a busy pub/club and enjoying myself with friends and family (Problem) I panic in crowds and get very edgy when I am closed in anywhere, never happened before AD.

And so the list continued until I got myself into such a state I didn't know if I was coming or going! I wonder when people are diagnosed with this awful disease, do they ever realise at the time the dramatic and damming changes that may happen. I know I didn't and I can't be on my own in this? A disease like this is so far reaching and has so many complications added to it, not only for the person involved but also their loved ones and friends.

Lives are changed!! Paths are altered forever, but amongst all this Mayhem and strife WE ADAPT!!!! IT'S WHAT WE DO!!!

We have to and we have to make the best of it!!! Life is for living, no matter what your Gender, religion or illness!! Life itself is a fight!! I have always taught my grandchildren; when they say "ITS NOT FAIR" I always say "LIFES NOT FAIR" but we make the most of it!!

So tomorrow is another day and long may we live it with hope, expectation and GUSTO !!!!!!

Just When You Think

Just when you think, all is ok,

And everything, is going your way,

When worries are small, almost minute,

And everything, seems ready to fruit,

Along comes fate, out of the blue,

To stand in your way, put you off cue,

Just when all, was going so well,

You find yourself back, wanting to yell,

Why does it always, seem to be me?

Always in chains and never feels free,

Always bad news, never the good,

No more the sunshine, always the flood,

We all have our limits, of what we can take,

Before we collapse, fall down and break,

All of my strength and hope comes from you,

Without family and friends, what am I to do,

So we will stay strong, together as one,

Until our fight is over and done

Life`s Gamble

Hello and today I would like to share with you something that happened whilst Elaine and I were out and about. I had woken a little bit "Cloudy" as I describe it and had already had a very disturbed night. The nightmares came thick and fast last night and are too horrific to publish, but after a bit of breakfast I explained to Elaine I had been stuck in long enough because of my Flu and needed some fresh air. Today being Saturday we always put the lottery on (Well, you can't win it unless you're in it can you??LOL) and what usually happens is Elaine plays the English Lottery and I (coming from good old Irish Stock and proud of it) play the Irish one. To place a bet on the Irish Lottery you have to place it on at a Bookmaker`s office. So, as Elaine was putting her lotto on at the local supermarket I always put mine on at the same time next door at the bookmaker's office, but this time it was different! As I walked into the bookies, something I have been doing once a week for many years, I looked around me and didn't recognise a thing!! It threw me for a couple of minutes and took me a few deep breaths to try and get my composure back. At this point you would have thought the first thing I would have done was to turn right round and walk out of the bookies and find Elaine, but I couldn't!!! I stood there, rooted to the spot with fear and I can honestly tell you it's one of the most frightening things I have ever felt! I felt so alone, so isolated, and even though things were going on around me as normal I just felt as if I had walked straight into a stranger's house straight off the street.

After how long, I really don't know, I managed to regain my composure and realised where I was, but unfortunately that wasn't the end of it. I had no trouble locating the tickets and filling it in but then came the question" What Day Is It" And no matter how hard I tried, no matter how hard I scanned the paper on the wall for a day and a date, nothing came !!!! I tried to think what I had done that morning "NOTHING" I tried to think what I had done yesterday "NOTHING" The Irish lottery can be played twice a week I thought, which day did I put it on last time ? "NOTHING"

By this time the feeling of helplessness and uselessness was covering my whole body and mind like a Velcro suit and I was becoming more panicky by the second!! I made for the nearest chair and sat down with such force you would have thought I had been dropped form a great height! Seconds, Minutes passed, I don't know which before a very bewildered man on the next table asked if I was ok. I nodded and he seemed reassured by this, until I blurted out "What day is it please? Well, you can only imagine the look of surprise on his face before he told me it was a Saturday and he got off his chair and hurried away from this "Weird" person who didn't even know what day it was. The feeling of rejection was unbearable and because I felt so humiliated by the whole thing I couldn't even blurt out my apologies and explanation of my illness of which I am certainly not ashamed of! Eventually I filled the date in on the ticket and placed my bet, and as I walked out of the shop, there was my "Angel" Elaine, waiting to meet me (always keeping her eyes out for me) As we got back into the car I explained to her everything, the feelings of despair, everything, and more importantly she listened and hung onto every word so she would know if it ever happened again. I have so much to be grateful for even though I have this terrible disease. This has never happened to me before in Public as it's very unusual for me to find myself anywhere without Elaine at my side, but as Optimistic and Bubbly as I am, I am also a realist and I know this is something that is part and parcel of this illness and is a definite downturn in my abilities.

I always promised you my friend that I would tell you all about the bad times and the good, and believe me this wasn't one of my better days, but, tomorrow is another day. It's another day to fight this illness all the way and another day to carry on fighting until they find a cure.

Life`s Lonely Dreams

Walking through life`s lonely dream`s,

Nothing`s real, or so it seems,

Familiar faces flashing by,

Never stopping to say "Hi"

Now they just ignore me,

I wish that they could see,

That because they don't say "Hi"

The tears that fill`s my eyes,

What have I to do?

To get this through to you,

I`m still me inside,

There`s no need to hide,

So the next time that we meet

I`m hoping we will greet,

Each other with a grin,

Let Friendships new begin

Looking Though the Fog

As the fog descends, which is so unkind?

Drifting through, all parts of my mind,

I start to stumble, stutter and fall,

Getting ever harder to recall,

What`s just been said, and just been done,

Unaware of where I am, is no fun,

Familiar places inside my head,

Seem to fade with such dread,

Voices louder, sound so loud,

Amidst this unforgiving cloud,

My "Angel" puts her hand in mime,

Always knowing when its time,

To "Take charge" and look after me,

Keeping me safe, so I will see,

Another day to live my life,

With my darling beautiful wife,

The dementia Demon came to call,

But when it did we stood tall,

Living our lives from day to day,

To survive another, is all we pray.

LOOKING BACK

So, here I am, at 53yrs of age with breathing problems and Alzheimer`s! If I had a pound each time people have said to me, "Try not to think about it" I would be a very rich man. And the times I have heard "You don't sound or look like you have Alzheimer's" is too many to count, but lately I have come to welcome such comments. Yes, it used to upset me and I would always make a point of telling them I was ill and the things that brings it to the surface. But I have noticed lately when someone says "You don't sound or look like you have Alzheimer's" I have replied "Thank you, it just shows the wonders of modern day medicine are working at their best! Depending on their reaction then depends on how I further the conversation and if they ask how it shows itself I will gladly tell them. I am very at peace with my diagnosis and what will be will be, but always in the back of my mind I know the dark days and cloudy days are always only a breath away.

As time strolls on and I look back at the fears and trembling I had about this disease I have decided that I am no less afraid of my diagnosis than I ever was, but what I am is more at ease with it. Am I coming to terms with my fate if they don't find a cure?? Maybe so, but the question is "how can this happen when I am convinced a cure is on the cards??? Very confusing! But as I have said before, this is what this awful disease does to you, its throws the very FIBRE`S of your life into doubt!!! It makes you think about (Or try to loll) everything you do or say before you do or say it! I dreamt about times gone past last night, of how I was again running up that cobbled back street making my way home after an afternoon on the park. I dreamt of my wonderful Grandmother who brought me up, sat in front of the range /oven/fire with cakes in the oven and socks drying on the top. Then there is the smell of homemade pea soup filling the house and the sound of a very crackling wireless playing in the background. I wake up, in tears and frustration as I realise I am back to reality with the fight of my life on my hands.

Do I miss my childhood? Of course I do, but as I turn over and see my beautiful wife sleeping, and realise this is the lady who has saved my life up to now and will do her upmost to do it again in the future as well as provided me with the most wonderful family in Gods kingdom.

Will I survive??? You bet!!!!!!!! And I would love for everybody to come along with me and watch me win this battle!!!

LOOKING TO THE FUTURE

Hiya, I would just like to share with you the good news and the good feeling I woke up with this morning. Yesterday we had a visit from the Social worker from our local memory clinic about possible housing needs for the future and more support for my darling Elaine. As a sufferer it was hard at first listening to Elaine and the social worker planning out my future care and possible end of life plans. The most important thing that came out of it was I and Elaine now have peace of mind knowing plans are made and arrangements for more support for Elaine is now in place and I meet my Community support worker tomorrow. All this has been playing on my mind lately and as you all know I always have and always will put my family first and now I know that Elaine will now be getting more rest and more "She" time I feel as if a huge weight is off my shoulders. But there are some sticking points LOL

It's the later on stages I can't really get my head around like washing and cleaning ECT by a stranger. Even before my illness if ever I was in hospital it has only ever been Elaine who has washed,, showered and shaved me ect. The thought of someone else doing this just frightens me to death and as much as I tell myself "I might not be too sure what is going on by that stage" It still petrifies me. On the one hand I don't want to become a burden for my family and on the other hand I can't imagine anybody else being there instead of Elaine. I can't be the only one who feels like this surely!! How many before me have felt the same but not mentioned it? Is this the reason for some people to behave totally out of character?? I wonder? What I do believe is plans like this must be talked about where and when possible right at the start of diagnosis. Because my family did this right from the start this has banished any demons about the disease they may have had and an acceptance follows quite quickly. (Pity most of my friends didn't do the same!!) I am not saying this will work for everyone but I thought it was worth sharing that it has worked for us.

91

As for the future, yes, plans are in place and the future is as about planned for, as this awful illness will allow it but as you know I am totally convinced that they will find a cure in my lifetime so it won't come to that will it??LOL LOL. Somebody asked me the other day if I was frightened of having Alzheimer`s and my honest answer was a great big YES!!!! BUT!! Ask me am I ashamed if it?? CERTAINLY NOT! In a very strange way, even though I have been burdened with this horrible disease I still feel blessed as I have been diagnosed young enough and early enough to hopefully make a difference for all sufferers out here for the betterment of treatment and reducing the stigma that's attached to this awful illness.

So it's onwards and upwards and the campaign goes on. Please, those who haven't joined me yet, please come and join me on my journey fighting this disease and together we will become victorious and the "Dementia Demon will be banished ONCE AND FOR ALL.

Party To Remember??

Yesterday was the leaving party for our youngest daughter and her family who are emigrating to Australia in eight days time. Family came from far and wide to give her a good send off. Aunties, uncles and cousin we hadn't seen for ages came to celebrate her new journey in life and her future success. As I sat there looking round, watching the children run riot playing dinosaurs and lions and marvelling at their imagination it suddenly hit me that everything I was watching seemed to be ten times magnified and much clearer. I found I was noticing things that I hadn't seen before like how much my grandchildren (who we see quite regularly) are growing up into their own little person`s. Their smiles and laughter seemed louder but much brighter. I could feel myself going just that bit taller every time they came over for a hug or said "Grandad, do you know what? It was oh so much simpler talking to them than it was the adults!! They take you as they see you; they still see the same old grandad that's always been there for them and never question when I am staring into space and in my own little world.

Wouldn't it be nice if everybody had the same outlook on Dementia as children do? Wouldn`t it be just great if people saw the person and not the illness just as children do? How is it they can come to terms with it so easily, yet some "Grown up adults can`t? We have much to teach our children to put them on the right path of life, but please remember

THEY HAVE MUCH TO TEACH US!!!

Sometime`s...........Just Sometime`s

Sometimes, just sometime`s, I wish something would go right! I wish that sometimes when I have a dream and want it to come true, it does!! Sometimes I just want to walk into the middle of a field away from all the noise and lie down to listen to the sound of nothing, smell the grass beneath me, and look up to the skies looking for the answer`s of the universe. Sometimes, just sometimes, I wish I couldn`t see the faces of people who are not here anymore flash in front of my eyes, or hear their voices shouting my name when I am alone in my thoughts. I wish I could have one night's sleep without the horrific Night terrors I have that keep my ANGEL Elaine awake most of the night, and probably half the neighbours! Sometimes, just sometimes, I wish I could look into the eyes of ALL my family and tell them everything is going to be ok and they have nothing to worry about. I wish I could take all their worry and woes away and protect them all as I did when they were little. I wish I could convince myself that all will be ok and a cure is just around the corner. I wish I had no need at all to take all the tablets I do or at the very least have a "DAY OFF" from talking them.

Sometimes, just sometimes, I wish I didn't have this depression that envelopes me some days like a concrete overcoat and I didn't have to hide my innermost fear and feelings for fear of upsetting some people, that I didn't have to smile my way through the day like a Cheshire cat instead of wanting to break down and cry like a baby, but because I am taking such a strong dose of Anti depressants this is just not possible. Sometimes, just sometimes, I wish I could spend a day and night without thinking of the future and what it may hold and living through every waking moment of this nightmare with Alzheimer's at every twist and turn, and people would stop saying "Try not to think about it" as well meant as that is, the truth is its impossible for me to do this. And finally, sometimes, just sometimes, I wish I didn't have this "GOD FORSAKEN DISEASE" Actually, that`s not true, I think about NOT having it ALL THE TIME! Maybe one day eh ?

94

The Fight Never Ends

Is it too soon to be talking of this?

Secretly remembering our first kiss,

Of how you will manage when I'm gone,

When my fight is finished, over and done,

I ask you this with tears in my eyes,

Trying to stifle a million cries,

Don't be so silly, you`ll outlast me!

Is always your answer, but please will you see,

I need to make sure that life will be kind,

And then you can rest and have peace of mind,

I need to say this before the AD,

Removes all my memories and steals them from me,

I didn't mean to make you cry,

Just want to be sure that you will get by,

You take hold of my hand and say" Listen to me"

Your going nowhere, why can't you see,

We are in this together, no matter how long,

Nobody`s singing their last song,

You have provided for us, all of your life,

And I`m proud to say that i am your wife,

We have wonderful kids, and grandchildren too,

All of them grateful for the kindness from you,

Then I say Shhh; please just let me say,

That when my time comes, no matter what day,

You shall remember, that very first kiss,

And how all our life has been absolute bliss,

And do me one favour, is my question to you,

When you look up, at a sky that's so blue,

Always remember, I will always love you,

And please say goodbye to all of my friends,

And always remember "The Fight Never Ends"

The Loneliness Of Dementia

Imagine this:

You have the most loving supportive family on your side and a wealth of friends that are with you every step of the way, yet you still feel like the loneliest person in the world. Quite a statement I know, but this is just one of the many ways dementia can make you feel. I am so lucky in many ways yet sometimes I feel as if nobody understands. I just know that's because it must be so very hard for them to put themselves in my shoes for a day. To be told that you have a brain wasting disease and at the moment there is no known cure is without doubt one of the worst things anybody can be told.

Sometimes I sit in my own little world, remembering things from days gone by. I remember my old house as a child and how I would walk up the backstreet hoping it was chips and pea soup for tea. As I walk in I can see dad sat there "In his chair" his feet in front of a roaring fire. As I look across the room I can see mum, busy at the cooker frying his sausages for tea, he always got his tea first as he was a hardworking man my mum always said to me. My wonderful grandmother would be there to visit bringing her homemade pies and cakes ready for the weekend feast. We didn't have much but we were very rarely hungry. Then I try to remember back to where I first met my "Angel "Elaine and tears fill my eyes. It's like trying to see though a very thick fog and every now and again the fog clears just a fraction and I see glimpses of Elaine and me walking hand in hand round the reservoir on a summers day, the smell of freshly cut grass and the blue clear still water with gentle ripples dancing across the top, all following each other in turn until they eventually run out of strength., reminding me that life is very similar and eventually we will all slow down.

My mind then shifts to try and remember later and suddenly I can hear children's voices, screaming with laughter and as I look through the fog I can just barely make out me pushing the swings in turn and trying to get them as high as possible. Then NOTHING!! A blackness envelopes my brain as I try with all my might to try and remember something else.

The pain is etched on my face as I screw my face up tight to try and remember just one more little thing!! But not tonight, that's it for tonight, memories gone, memories of times gone past which are slowly but surely being taken from me as I sit here, how cruel this disease is.

As I look across the room I see my darling Elaine giggling at something on the television and my mood lifts, but the loneliness stays in the pit on my stomach. How can a man or woman have so much yet feel so desperately lonely? The only answer is because of Dementia and the fear of losing the battle against it. Not only does the dementia win but it takes with it, all your precious memories, hopes dreams and locks them up in a very dark place.

Well not my memories, and not my dreams and hopes for the future. I won't allow it, I just WONT!!!!

THE REALITY OF ALZHEIMERS

I knew something was wrong as I sat in my chair and felt as though somebody was trying to push me down into the Abyss. I usually call this my "Concrete Overcoat" as depression meets Alzheimer's and clashes together like a deafening thunderclap and clouds my brain into thinking there is nothing left in the world that is good" A bold statement you may think but this is what happens when out of the blue the depression that goes with the knowledge of having such a horrid disease which has already claimed the lives of some of my family.

This is the reality of having an Alzheimer's diagnosis.

So there I sat, in my chair, trying to remember all the good things I have in my life, my family, my friends and my abilities to try and carry on, but nothing but blackness and despair runs through my tormented mind. I look across at my "Angel" wife Elaine, she know something is wrong immediately by the look in my eyes. She crosses the room and whilst standing, cradles my head into her lap, just as my wonderful grandmother used to do when I was but a child." Everything will be ok you know" she whispers to me while stroking my hair, but at this moment in time, nothing can convince me. Maybe it's a culmination of turning fifty three, and reading a letter from my clinical Phshycolgist I received a day or so ago when she asked me to help her write a paper about being told at such an early age you have Alzheimer`s. I remember the statement "I was there when you were diagnosed and saw how you looked." Maybe I had become complacent in trying to forget I was suffering from this awful thing. All this together must have triggered something and I couldn't see past anything at all at this moment.

I AM SO SCARED!!!!! MORE SCARED THAN I HAVE EVER BEEN IN MY LIFE!!!

There, I have said it now, it's out in the open, and this is the raw reality of what it's like to be told you have early onset of Alzheimer's at the age of fifty!! I`m scared, I'm scared for my family, I'm scared for what I may turn into but most of all I am scared to die !! I have wrote this just to try and show you wonderful people who look after people like me what must be going through the minds of so many people in my position and also must have gone through the minds of those who are further down the line than me. This is the truth of this unforgiving disease.

I know it's not my usual upbeat post but Dementia has many faces, some I am good at hiding at, and some I have no control over.

"Please God they will find a cure someday"

As the night passed and I drifted off to sleep eventually after much reassurance from my darling wife, a million dreams came rushing through my mind, all dark and all to horrific to describe here. The following morning we both arose, very tired but yet feeling we have survived yet another battle whilst knowing there will be many more to come. But with Elaine, my family and my friends by my side I just know that all will be ok.

"Until the "Concrete Overcoat "calls again

Time and Tide

Just like the saying "Time and Tide wait for no man (or woman) "then neither does Alzheimer`s. Every morning when I awake I am so thankful I have survived another night. They are so much longer these days and yes the days seem shorter. I remember a time when if I woke at two of three in the morning I used to think "WOW" is it only that time, more sleep for me!!! Nowadays because I am up and down on average six/seven times a night when I look at the clock I am wishing that is daylight and I can get up! I don't think it's so much the "more" getting up as this usually just makes me more tired but I really do think that it's a couple of things, please, let me (TRY LOL) and explain.

I think because it's a fatal disease, and please, let's make no mistake about this, unless a cure is found, it certainly is, then the fear of dying is implanted somewhere deep inside my head and being up and about in the daylight hours is my way of knowing I am ok, I have survived another day to fight this awful disease. Another way of looking at it is because I am so determined to win this battle I am in; I don't want to miss a single second of this wonderful life!!!! And part of winning this battle is accepting my disease and trying to raise as much awareness about it as I can.

When I speak at conferences ECT I always say the following.

"I cannot understand why "Dementia doesn't get the same funding as the other big Charities such as the Heart foundation or Cancer UK" Did you know that Dementia only gets an EIGHTH of the funding the other two charities get from the Government in the UK!"! How is this possible? "I have met someone who had a brain tumour and survived, I have met people who had cancer and survived and I know many people who have had heart attacks and survived BUT?????????

101

I have never met anybody who has had Alzheimer`s and survived!!!!

Maybe this is why I don't sleep as well as I did?

Maybe my strength and desire to survive is so strong I don't want to sleep in?

Maybe I just don't want to miss a thing and cherish as much as I can from this life?

But do you know what I think??

I think it's because I know I have so much left to do and so much more to give!! I am just not ready yet for throwing in the towel! So I am afraid you are going to have to put up with me a little bit longer yet (Hopefully a lot longer LOL) and I am SURE, together, we will see that all elusive cure developed!! Have faith my friends and remember, where there is HOPE life will always find a way

TIME TO LISTEN

Taken from the song Vincent,

"Now I understand, what you tried to say to me"

"And how you suffered for your sanity,

How you tried to set them free"

They would not listen, they would not know how"

Perhaps they`ll listen now"

Have there ever been any more powerful or evocative words spoken about mental illness than these?? I think not. And if you relate it to anybody who has been unfortunate enough to be touched by this vile disease of dementia whether it is by suffering from it or knowing someone who does/have it? Then the words truly hit home.

I believe the time is NOW!! I believe that OUR time is NOW!! We must be listened to, from the streets of people who snigger or are appalled at the word of DEMENTIA right up to the houses of Parliament and Downing Street. It's almost every day it's been researched and reported that Dementia will be a huge problem in the near future (as if it isn't big enough now!) And yet it's still a postcode lottery regarding who gets the drugs that could possibly stave off this awful disease and give people not only like myself but thousands of others a glimmer of hope until a cure is finally found as I do believe it will be one day soon. But that day is not soon enough for some who are being refused treatment every day because of where they live or the cost of medicine!! I have campaigned the best way I know for a while now to raise awareness and lately I am not only surprised but appalled that when I have e mailed some of the "BIG GUNS" who shall remain nameless they have not even had the courtesy to reply to my offer of help or acknowledged that there is a problem.

I am not blaming governments, I am not blaming health workers and I am certainly not blaming Doctors whose hands are tied by faceless officials! But I do believe that this is OUR time to STAND UP AND BE HEARD!! All I want to do is get those who shall not be named, or can't be named to listen to what's being said. Just listen to our story of loved ones lost unnecessarily and the pain sorrow and millions of tears shed every day because of this horrible thing called Dementia

PLEASE JUST LISTEN !!

Times and Places

Hello, well it was great to see all my friends in Bolton and also visit Blackpool. The Hotel was fantastic and if anybody wants to know anything about it please just ask. The one thing I did discover whilst travelling was my concept of time and places had worsened considerably. For a while now Elaine has been telling me that sometimes when she has only been in the kitchen for a few minutes I have come in behind her asking why she has been in there for hours? Whilst we were away Elaine was explaining to people we met that we had been living in Torquay for the last twelve years, this come as a complete surprise to me !!!! A lot of explaining was needed when I questioned this and also an explanation was needed of my condition to my "New friends" as they looked quite bemused as to why I didn't know! Twelve Years??? I kept repeating to myself, how can that be ? As hard as I tried to remember I couldn't, and the feeling is as horrible as anyone can imagine. Twelve years? Where had they gone?? What had happened in all that time??

I can remember being a manager at Focus DIY but that seems like only yesterday, and I have a little recollection of other things, but the rest, at the moment is a complete mystery. If you can imagine this, my memories are like the old Cine Film that used to flicker past very quickly and I only get a glimpse of what has happened in the past. It's very frightening and also very soul destroying. On the way home last night for safety reasons we stopped for a rest about half way home but as Elaine was telling me this morning we stopped for a good 45 mins where I am convinced it was a quick toilet break, coffee and away!!! The time thing with me seems to work both ways, sometimes its quick and sometimes it's like time stands still. Either way it`s just another sign that things are deteriorating and I suppose if I was honest about it even I can now see a downward turn.

So, the RACE **IS NOW ON!!!**

It's now April and September is only about 5 months away!! Taking that into consideration and also my scan today (I have also had a few more worrying problems in that dept the last 24 hours) I am more determined now than ever to make **Dementia Awareness Day the Biggest dementia awareness day event of the yearly calendar!!** And I promise as always to do what I can for as long as I can to make this happen!!!!

Tough Week

I can honestly say this has been one of the toughest weeks of my life. Certain things about my Ad have been working their way into my life, IE- Mood swings, and outbursts of temper (never even heard of before) and believe it or not a major Tantrum!! I have eight beautiful grandchildren and I know a tantrum when I see one, let alone have one! This completely threw my darling wife Elaine and ended in floods of tears from both of us. All this with my illness of heart failure and AD, and Elaine worrying herself sick and wham! Some would say no wonder there was a bit of stress and upset but things have been thrown at us before, with such a big family these things always are, but this was different. I was different! No longer was i the laid back, positive optimist i always am. It was like i was so different and the thing is most of it i can't remember! I rely on my angel wife so much and to see her so upset really cuts deep with me. I want to be so strong for my family as i have always been before but i am now very afraid of not coping very well in these times of great worry. I have made an appointment to see my specialist and my CPN as i was advised this would be the best next step for me. Is this the beginning of the End??

NO SIR!! Not if I have anything to do about it!! I will fight this horrid illness right to the end and never give up hope that someday, before it's too late, they will find a cure, then i will laugh in the face of AD and say " I`m the one that got away! The support i get from all my friends is wonderful and even though i might be taking a few days off to try and settle my families worries about their concerns, you will ALL never be far from my thoughts, thank you so much,

LOOKING THROUGH THEIR EYES

Try looking through your children's eyes,

And tell me what you see,

It matters not how old they are,

They`re so special to you and me,

Has my illness changed their lives?

In any way at all,

Or is it Musketeer time,

All shouting "ONE FOR ALL!"

As I look into their eyes,

Trying to read between the lines,

Do they ever cast their minds?

Back to better times,

When days were always sunny,

And laughter could be heard,

And there was never ever a mention,

Of that dammed dementia word,

Does it now cloud their lives?

And everything they do,

Or have they taken it in their stride,

Respecting me and you,

I sometimes read their pain,

Hidden behind their eyes,

And wish that it would disappear,

And stifle all their cries,

Yes I have The Alzheimer's,

And a failing heart,

But I would never change a day,

From the very start,

So to family and my friends,

We will walk as one,

Until our day is over,

And the setting of the sun

Trying To Remember

Hiya, we recently came back from a two day jaunt in Minehead last weekend and even though a good time was had it was tinged with a little sadness because of my failing memory. Unknown to me we had holidayed in Somerset four times in the last two years and some of them I have no recollection whatsoever. It's so frustrating!!! I cannot put into words how frustrating this illness is. Not only does it eat away at your self esteem but robs you of your most precious memories!! I listen transfixed at the tales what my "Angel" Elaine tells me and what we (or should I say I LOL) got up to and the feeling of "Wishing I was there" is overwhelming but made even worse so by the knowledge that I was, but can't remember a B****Y thing! All this seems to build up inside and sometimes without warning it explodes into a rage of frustration so much so I have to remove myself from the room I am in and put my headphones on, and with my music playing in my ears, it has, up to now, calmed me down.

This is one of the ways I try to deal with it but there must be so many people a lot farther down the line than me that can't find that escape valve and at times like this I think it's so important to remember that it's just this horrid illness and not the real person inside. I have lost count the amount of times I have asked "WHY ME???" and wished all was back to normal, but it's not, and unless they find a cure it never will be. This also adds to any frustration I may already have so sometimes I feel as if I am in a never ending circle of desperation and depression. Can you imagine not being able to remember the things you have been told you have done?? Also knowing that at the moment things could only get worse?

I do use the word "Could" because deep down in my heart I feel with all my being that a cure will come soon and it's that "HOPE!!! That keeps me going. I am convinced that some who are a lot worse off than me also HOPE and pray deep down to be freed one day from this awful prison of Alzheimer's we are stuck in. The knowing is an awful thing but at the moment I can relate to it and write my feelings down. Can you imagine what it must be like to think as I do but are unable to convey that to the world?? It's one of my worst nightmares and I promise with all my heart I will carry on doing what I can while I can and for as long as I can.

Under Stress

As I sit here on this sunny day,

With my hospital appointment only hours away,

I start to think of what I've done,

During my life, how far I have come,

The clock is ticking in so many ways,

What's to happen in these coming days?

It's going to be tough, I can't deny this,

Not something to remedy, with a lingering kiss,

All through my life I've faced many things,

With all its worries and troubles it brings,

But for most of my years, stood by my side,

Has been my wonderful wife, I'm bursting with pride,

Thinking how she has helped, through the dark days,

And how she has chased my demons away,

So why does it feel so different this time,

Have I done something wrong, stepped out of line?

Whatever it is I know we will face,

The troubles ahead, and with such grace,

What lays ahead, in this future of ours?

Will be revealed, in a few hours,

Whatever it is, I promise to fight,

Of my survival I will not lose sight,

With all of my family and friends by my side,

I have nothing to fear, nothing to hide

Wandering Mind

Hiya, we have just come back from one of the most beautiful places on earth, a little village within Torquay called "Cockington Village" It's a place where time has stood still now for over three hundred years and apart from the red post boxes and ice cream signs you would swear you have been transported back to another time. The walk up to the village is among countryside and a babbling brook which always looks so welcome when the sun shines. The birds sing loud and clear and sheep can be heard baying in the fields. Admittedly with everything that has been going on this past couple of weeks my mind started to wander somewhat, and as I watched Elaine and my Granddaughter throwing sticks in the river to race, I suddenly felt very mortal and very vulnerable.

The past couple of days I have been experiencing a few low abdominal aches and pains which I hadn't noticed before. My mind races at a thousand miles an hour when this happens as I always doubt if they are real or not!! Is this yet another present from the dreaded Alzheimer's disease? Am I imagining these pains? As I do other things like noises/voices ECT? Or is it what I fear most? Only the scans next Thursday will reveal that, but having a diagnosis of AD like I do, this is what happens, it throws your whole outlook on life and sanity into question! When I was diagnosed with heart failure, to be honest it never really sank in how ill I was. When I was diagnosed with Alzheimer's, once I started on the Ebixa Tablets and "Came back from the brink" as I call it, as time has passed I must admit to becoming a little complacent about it, almost laughing at it (Is this such a bad thing though? A question for another day me thinks!) But they do say things come in three`s don't they? And if this is what I fear most, bowel or bladder cancer, then it will throw up a whole new set of questions that will need answering as quickly as possible depending on the results.

Am I frightened? Yes, I am petrified; can I stop thinking about it? No I cannot!! But can I try to make the most of my time whatever the outcome

YES I CAN!!!!!!!!!!

Yes my friends, I am frightened, of course I am, I couldn't imagine anyone not being. As strange as it sounds you would think that having Alzheimer's already would be frightening enough, and you would be right. But this is a different kind of frightened; this might be a different enemy that causes more pain and doesn't move the goal posts, it's just either wins or not, simple as that!!! I always believe that a cure for Alzheimer's is very close and soon to be available to all, I have to believe this because of my families sake, but there is always a chance that this other disease might have taken such a hold that there is nothing that can be done. This is by far my biggest fear!! These are the things that are racing through my mind and as I have always been honest about the way I feel about my Alzheimer's, then this is no different, because it's still me, I am still Norrms no matter what!!

And this has only made me feel more determined to go on "THE PEPSI BIG ONE" (big dipper in Blackpool) next week LOL LOL

We shall be leaving early tomorrow so please , will everybody have a fantastic week and please stay safe, I will miss each and every one of you and don't forget to advertise "Dementia Awareness Day " where ever and whenever you can,

What Of The Future?

Hiya, I was asked yesterday if ever I thought about the future as I am always saying this disease dictates that we live every day as it comes to make the best of a bad situation, slight understatement there but I am sure you know what I mean. I suppose the answer is yes I have thought about it but not for a while now. The first thing that always comes to mind when I think of my future is my family. How will they manage? Will they be ok? What about their future? I have always said my main aim is to make sure Elaine "My Angel" is secure in every possible way to ensure a bright and happy future without me, this I can say, with peace of mind, has been done. Then my thoughts go to my children who are all grown up now and making their way in the world as they should, and as I think of them I grow a little taller as I am so proud of them all. We walked many roads together, both rocky roads and even roads but together we walked them and got there in the end. It was not only character building for them but as anyone knows who have children it's also character building for the parents as well!!

Then, of course without exception are my grandchildren, all nine of them!! The eldest are three girls, 18yrs, 14yrs (Going on 30yrs loll) and eleven (the clever one LOL) The one thing I have always said since finding out I had this terrible disease is my aim in life was to see my three girls "Walking down the aisle" and I would be a very happy man. This still stands as I intend fighting this demon called "dementia" to the very end. The very thought of me not being there for their biggest day fills me with dread and believe me it will be worth fighting for. The other six grandchildren are boys ranging from eight downwards!! So as you can see, even with my optimistic outlook I might be pushing it a little to be there for their stag nights!!LOL Still you never know?? I am so immersed in helping my grandchildren to grow up into the adults I know they can be I don't often think that far into the future, but when I do

I must admit it takes two different roads. The first road is either watching or walking my granddaughters down the aisle, holding on to them so tight, I don't really want them to get married but I know they must, but be guaranteed, tears of happiness will flow! The other road is much different; it's one of fear for the future and the unknown. I read each and every day how you brave carers deal with the most horrific situations and how much you give every time you are asked without question. The things I read are real and uncompromising accounts at what this awful disease does to people, and their loved ones/carers ECT. Is this my future?? Is this is what to come?? Will I be such a burden for my family? Do all these things go through the heads of people in my position? Surely it must do but as I have said before, we get very very good at hiding things and especially our feelings. So back to the original question "Do I think of the future?? I suppose the honest answer is no, not that much, as when I do it can take me down either road which is such a roller coaster of emotions the end event can be just as bad as each other. Unfortunately this does raise the question "What's it like to live day to day without a clear future in mind" But that's a question for another day.

As a footnote the only other thing I think, pray and hope for is a cure to become a reality to end this awful uncertainty and banish this Godforsaken disease forever.

When It All Becomes Too Much

The last couple of mornings I have been woken by my "ANGEL" Elaine telling me I have been weeping in my sleep. This has happened two days together, this morning included and the reason I want to share this with you is this. When times are hard "You Are There" When trouble flare`s "You Are There" When "THEY" Don't understand "You Are There" and when I feel like no one care`s "You Are There" Who am I talking about????

ALL YOU WONDERFUL CARER`S AND LOVED ONES OUT THERE!!!!

I dread to think where we would be without you!! Today I wasn't at my best as the nightmare`s the last few days have taken their toll, but off to the garden centre we went today anyway because Elaine, just like all you wonderful carers out there knew it was "The Right thing to do" It took me out of the situation and took me away from surroundings that can become ever decreasingly smaller some days. Don't get me wrong, I love my little house but sometimes I can feel the walls closing in, but, as carers (Caregivers) you know that don't you? This illness shows itself in many ways that others can't understand (But you carers do)

When we arrived at the garden centre Elaine just gave me a little nudge and a cheeky wink and said "Shhh, a little quieter please" because apparently I was talking very loud!!LOL Within minutes my mood changed and I just felt as if it didn't matter what I did or said I was always in the wrong!! I started to stumble over my words, I felt so insecure and I was walking as if I was drunk. The clouds came thick and fast and the day was going downhill fast!! When I say clouds, for anybody who doesn't know it's when my Alzheimer's is getting worse and it's as if I am looking at life through a cloud of fog, or trying to look through net curtains but just can't quite make out what's going on. This can sometimes last, minutes, hours or days, this disease know no rules or regulations!!!

118

There is no "Fair Play "in this illnesses dictionary!! Its an all out war between me and my Alzheimer's!!!! But through all this, through all the raised voices/ stumbling/ slurred speech and nods/ winks and a lot of tutting and shaking of heads by other members of the public

YOU CARERS/CAREGIVERS AND LOVED ONES ARE THERE AND YOU CARE!!!!

You stay with us and you look after us, you hold our hands and talk to us in a calming voice that reassures us and tells us that no matter what is happening or whatever happens in the future you will always be at our side telling us everything is going to be ok.

There are no words in the worlds dictionary/whatever language you speak or where ever you live in the world that could express the heartfelt gratitude we , as People have with Dementia have, for all of you wonderful people out there who give so much yet expect so little in return!! Thank you just doesn't seem enough somehow but it's all I have at the moment so

THANK YOU SO MUCH EACH AND EVERY ONE OF YOU!!!

A Story OF HOPE, TRUTH

AND EVENTUAL

TRIUMPH

When my husband was 48 years old, I began to notice a change in his behavior and moods; he was signed off work with depression and prescribed anti depressants. Shortly after that his father died and everyone assumed that this was the cause of his erratic behavior. He was also good at masking what was happening in front of others and I know that some of his family thought I was being silly when I enquired about any history of AD in the family.

After 15 months of him being treated for depression, I had had enough and insisted on going with him to his next GP appointment. I told the doctor I was not happy with the diagnosis and wanted him to see a consultant and have any relevant tests done to get a proper diagnosis. He was sent an appointment with a Parkinson's consultant who diagnosed Parkinson Disease and he was given new medications. After several months of this I asked to speak to the consultant and told him I felt it wasn't the right diagnosis still. He examined my husband and did more tests and finally we received a diagnosis of Lewy Body Dementia and he was given a cocktail of drugs to take.

Initially these helped his condition but over time his health began to deteriorate- his cognitive skills declined massively, he suffered terrifying hallucinations, his speech was very hard to understand and his mobility gradually got less and less. After being hospitalized a couple of times with infections which sped up the progress of his condition, we had to move home to a ground floor flat as he could no longer manage stairs, in fact he could only go outdoors in his wheelchair, needed support moving around indoors, washing, dressing and eating.

He would sleep for a great deal of the day, became physically and verbally aggressive and when not asleep would sit in his chair staring at the wall with no interest in reading, watching TV or making conversation. It was a very grim and upsetting time for us all. I had more or less been told by a doctor on his discharge from hospital the last time that this was the progress of his condition and that it wouldn't get any better than this- and at this point he was only 55 years old. Being unable to go out much as he couldn't be left alone, I spent a lot of time online, and it was online that I first 'met' Norman Mc Namara- a meeting which has turned our lives around! He spoke openly about his illness as he fights to raise awareness of dementia and remove the stigma surrounding it, and mentioned a drug his consultant had prescribed him which had made such a difference to his health. This drug was Ebixa- I began to read up about Ebixa to see if it was something that could help us and decided to ask the Parkinson's consultant to prescribe it. As his next appointment approached I started to get excited at the thought of a drug that would slow the progress of this dreadful illness but was thwarted when the consultant said he didn't think there were any benefits in my husband taking it and wouldn't prescribe it for him.

But I wasn't going to take this lying down! The following week my husband had an appointment with his psychiatric consultant and I determined to ask her about Ebixa. I gave her all the information I had about it, told her of Norrms experience taking it and she said she would look into it and get back to me via the CPN if she thought it would be worth trying. Time dragged on until eventually we got a call saying he could have a 3 month trial of Ebixa, closely monitored to see if it was helping. I have to say at this point that she had to argue her case for the trial long and hard before it was agreed to, and I really appreciate all the effort she made on our behalf.

After just 2 weeks of taking it, my husbands speech became clearer with better volume (before he spoke in virtually a whisper) and we were able to have good conversations. Over the next few weeks, he continued to improve, sleeping better at night, watching TV and taking an interest, picking up a book to read. His mobility improved, he was able to wash and dress himself with a little bit of assistance. His cheerful, cheeky demeanour returned and an increased enjoyment of life compared to the apathy he had displayed previously. After 10 weeks of taking Ebixa, he stepped out of our flat for the first time since we moved here (10 months ago) and we went for a walk, using just a walking stick for support! Ever since then we go out daily for a walk, building up the distance we go to build up his strength a bit at a time.

He can now even manage to fasten the buttons on his shirt, something he hadn't been able to do for many months. We have now been told he can stay on Ebixa long term as it has not only slowed down the progress of his illness, it has quite amazingly reversed several of the symptoms. Last week we went back for an appointment to the Parkinson's clinic, where unfortunately the consultant who wouldn't prescribe Ebixa was on annual leave- but the Parkinson's nurse was astounded at how well my husband is, as were several other members of staff, who all came out to see him and how well he is doing! In fact I was told that one of the nurses was crying, she was so happy to see him so well My hope is that now the psychiatric consultant and the Parkinson's nurse have firsthand knowledge of the difference this medication can make to a persons life that they will consider it when meeting with other patients who may benefit and give them the chance we have been lucky enough to have. I am aware that Ebixa won't help everyone but as it only takes a 3 month trial to see if it will be effective I believe that everyone should have the opportunity to see if it works for them, and can give them back some quality of life.

Our lives have improved dramatically since we learnt about Ebixa, and managed to get it prescribed for my husband- and for that I can only thank my wonderful friend Norrms who is doing such a great job of raising awareness of dementia-he is truly my hero!

When the Clouds Roll In

It was 6-15pm last Saturday as I looked at my watch and smiled at something Elaine had said, she always makes me laugh. By 6-30 the clouds had come thick and fast in my head, descending so fast and taking me completely by surprise. Normally I can feel the pressure building up in my head but not this time. I was watching something on TV, I can't remember what now, when all of a sudden nothing made sense and everything around me became louder and distorted. I squinted as I strained to look at the television and tried to comprehend what was on at the time but nothing came. My frustration got the better of me as I put both hands on my head and pulled at my hair. Such are the devastating effects of this awful disease! I knew then this wouldn't pass soon and as the night drew on I became even more restless and incredibly tired. I asked to go to bed at seven fifteen but Elaine say's it too early, by seven forty five my head is dropping and my eyes are closing. Elaine puts the big light on to keep me awake but it's no use and by eight thirty I am tucked up in bed, knowing the nightmares are waiting to greet me.

After what only seems like an hour or so but is actually eight hours and a half I try to get out of bed and go to the bathroom but I struggle as I stumble into walls down the corridor as I feel as if I am drunk. Elaine is out of bed in an instant!! She looks so tired as I have no recollection of what antics I may have got up to during the night and when I ask her she just says I wasn't "That Bad? During the day I stumble over my words just like I did before I was taking the Ebixa and I am petrified I have taken a step backwards instead of my usual positive step forwards. But thankfully, as the day draws on I seem to get a little better and the clouds that invaded my mind and clouded my visions and speech start to disperse and fade away as if nothing had happened.

This is just one of many different episodes I will experience along this hard and rocky road of Alzheimer's disease. This disease has no shame, it creeps up when it wants to, and just to let you know he is still here and can take parts of your brain and memories whenever he wants to. He pushes you that little bit further every time just to see how much you can take!! Well, my unwanted enemy, I can still take much more!!! And it will take more than a couple of cloudy days, loss of speech and rubber legs syndrome to get the better of me!!!! I feel as if I have survived another battle with this Godforsaken illness and I live to fight another day! But deep in the back of my mind I can`t help feeling that he has stolen just a little bit more from my memories, we will have to wait and see, wont we ?

When Was The Last Time

Can I ask you something? When was the last time you asked a Dementia sufferer "What they wanted" When was the last time you asked a dementia sufferer "What would you like to see changed for the better so as to make sure you are getting as much out of life as you so richly deserve?. When was the last time you actually sat them down, looked them in the eye and asked how they felt their treatment was going? No, I don't mean ask the carer or loved one who has just done a 100hour week+ and been up all night and practically on their knees with exhaustion what they think? No I mean actually asked the person who has dementia what do they think?

Whilst I know there are many dementia sufferers who are at such a late stage in this disease that this is not possible, but I also know of many more that still have a voice and still have a life. Its people like these who need to be heard. These are the people who can and will make a change to the way things are in the health service and private service regarding Dementia and how it's perceived. It will also rid this awful disease of the stigma and mystery that's attached to it. This kind of Stigma is engrained in peoples mind because dementia sufferers up to now have been underestimated and in a lot of cases been spoken "On Behalf Of" We only have to look at the hospitals up and down the country and the startled look in a lot of nurses' eyes on being told the patient had dementia!!! This is not the nurse's fault, WHY?? They have not yet been trained to deal with this kind of thing from day one. YET!! They are highly trained to treat others with various illnesses with the dignity and respect they deserve. Does this mean Dementia is not treated as an actual illness just like the others?

I received a letter today from the "House Of Commons" informing me that the questions I have asked regarding the care of "Younger Early Onset" and the age limit for admissions' has been sent to the minister of health and I will receive a full explanation soon (Here`s hoping?) Next month I am going to the Dementia Uk conference in Bournemouth and then attending an Alzheimer's South West Dementia Strategy meeting in Bridgewater where I will be asking the same questions.

Who will be there?

Who will be there

For my end of life care,

How will they know?

I want it just so,

We've had this discussion

Me and my wife,

Of how I want things

At the end of my life,

Don't say that!

Some people say,

But how will they know,

At the end of the day,

How I want things,

If we don't talk,

To get it all ready

For my last walk,

I wish more people

Would talk about this,

Before they share

Their very last kiss,

So who will be there?

At my end of life care,

My family and friends,

Will all be there

Why is it?

Why is it that when we are young, the end of September is an age away from Christmas? Yet as we get older we think that at this time of year Christmas is just around the corner? Maybe I think too much?? LOL but my consultant did say to me "Use it or lose it" when he first diagnosed me two years ago. Such things go through my head a lot more these days and I do find myself thinking back to boyhood days.

Those days seemed much simpler then, harder? YES! But simple

If there is one thing to say about this awful disease is usually some of your best and earliest memories are usually the last to go. As you can imagine this throws up such a confusion of emotions as I like to think that I have many many happy memories of my life early and lately (what I can remember) the sheer thought of forgetting my darling wife and my family fills me with such dread some days that I actually shake with fear. I have always had this fear, even before my diagnosis that I will wake up one day, alone; all by myself and all my life has just been a dream. Then only to be told two years ago that there is a strong possibility this is going to actually happen!! Most of my memories eaten away by this unforgiving disease of the brain until all I see are my boyhood memories, if I am lucky. All this drives me on to do as much as I can, whilst I can, for as long as I can as I quite flatly refuse to lie down to this illness or roll over.

Yesterday Elaine and me attended out Memory Cafe we volunteer at and I was asked to say a few words about my illness (me? a few words? Are you kidding me??LOL LOL) So trying to raise awareness I said that at one time the word "Cancer" was only whispered about or called the big "C" Then of course we had HIV or "Aids" which seemed to be only talked about in corners or not at all.

Now both subjects are talked about openly and honestly. WHY??? Because we brought it to the forefront of people's attention! We advertised the fact that it's just an illness and not something to be scared of! We stood up to it and admitted more needed to be done to combat awful diseases like this. Because of this, people listened, Government listened and the generosity of human beings came to the forefront! They stood side by side to be counted and made their donations which are needed and are so welcome to fund research and hopefully one day a cure. The result is what we have today. Millions of pounds being donated by the government for research and the words Cancer or HIV used as commonly as any other word.

So what of the word Dementia? Why, in this day and age is it still only whispered about? Why do Governments plough more money into one disease than another when they are all equally devastating? The answer is quite simple when you think about it! If it wasn't for those wonderful people campaigning about the diseases mentioned and driving the message forward that more awareness needed to be raised then the general public would still be talking about Cancer and HIV in whispers! Does the same not apply to the word DEMETIA?? Of course it does!! And by raising awareness as much as possible about DEMENTIA and all its problems can, and will, benefit Dementia sufferers now and for the future. So come on guys, it worked for other diseases and I hope and pray it will work for this disease in my lifetime and a cure will be found.

HELP RAISE AWARENESS.

Without Warning

Usually, when I have a bad night there is some kind of warning, cloudy brain, on edge, losing concentration easily, but last night was the exception. I know I have had a very stressful week and will continue to have until the results of my tests are through (I lost a little more blood through my urine today which hasn't helped! But I went to bed quite relaxed after listening to my music for an hour before I sleep as I usually do. But last night was different. I remember waking just at the end of my scream, and when I say scream, it was more like a wounded animal in so much pain, GOODNESS KNOWS what the neighbours must think!! I was sweaty, shaking and trembling all over, my eyes went straight to my "Angel" Elaine who had a hold on me as tight as I have ever experienced before!! This isn't normal!!!! I shouted and started to shake!!

It took me quite a while to calm down and much gentle talking from Elaine who was hugging me and stroking my hair, I felt as if I was 6 years old again. The fear of what's to come or what might be to come washed over me time and time again, and with the added extra worry of this recent episode the feeling of complete helplessness is one I wouldn't wish on anybody!! The sheer enormity of my situation seemed to crash and burn inside my head time and time again. Dear God!! I thought what I have ever done to deserve this?? Heart Failure, Alzheimer's and now POSSIBLY something else, why can't I just be left alone to live my life just like anybody else?? I felt so sorry for myself at that particular moment, I felt so alone yet surrounded with love, I felt utter despair enter my soul. Then Elaine took my hand in hers and she whispered "I love you"

Never has these three words sounded so sweet, never has those three words sounded as reassuring as they did last night and they are three words I could never tire of. I raised my head off the pillow and managed a wry smile. I looked in my Angels eyes and saw hope and compassion rushing towards me and my spirits lifted. Deep down I know the fear that is behind those wonderful beautiful eyes, and Elaine knows that I know, but it's one of those things we don't talk about, as we only try to concentrate on the positive`s. As I drifted off in to what I would call I Fitful sleep, somewhere deep down I knew that with my Angel, my family and all my friends by my side I can face anything, and I fully intend to! So do your best Alzheimer`s, I wouldn't credit you with calling you Mister!!! And if there is anything else wrong with me, I know that whatever it is we will all face it together, with Pride, with Dignity but most of all, with HOPE!!!!

WHY ME?

A thousand times this has been asked,

Especially taking my Doctor to task,

What have I done that`s so very wrong,

To be punished like this for so long,

Most other illness`s come and go,

This one stays as we all know,

It lives within to the bitter end,

Always an enemy, never a friend,

It has no voice, the demon that grows,

Where it comes from no one knows,

It strips you of your very being,

Always there, always seeing,

Causing destruction all around,

Doing all this without a sound,

Taking you away, from your way of life,

Your dignity, children and also your wife,

What is this silent monster I talk about?

What's so quiet with no need to shout?

It's the curse of Dementia, and all it entails,

Raising its ugly head, it never fails,

To bring such sorrow, upset and pain,

Hiding the sunshine and bringing the rain,

To a life which was once so full,

Always bright and never dull,

But heed my waning bringer of doom,

I promise you this, one day soon,

You will be beaten, over and done,

And out again will come the sun,

I promise this with all my heart,

And once again my life will start,

I will live again, just you wait and see

And never again will you hang over me.

Best wishes, Norrms and family xxxxxxxxxxxxxxx

Few Words from Norrms

Hiya everybody, I do hope you have enjoyed this book and it has helped you understand this awful disease a little bit more. I want this book not only to help those with Dementia but also all those who are touched by this disease and all those professionals who, I hope, will be just that little better off from listening to someone who actually has the disease.

May your God always walk with you,
All my love,
Norrms, Elaine "MY ANGEL" and family xxx

E Mail   normmc1957@yahoo.co.uk

9595768R0008

Made in the USA
Charleston, SC
28 September 2011